Natural Healing for Headaches

Natural Healing for Headaches

High-Powered Cures for Ending Pain

Eva Urbaniak, N.D.

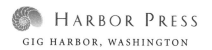 HARBOR PRESS

GIG HARBOR, WASHINGTON

Library of Congress Cataloging-in-Publication Data

Urbaniak, Eva, 1953-
    Natural healing for headaches: high-powered cures for ending pain /Eva
    Urbaniak.
    p.   cm.
    Includes bibliographical references and index.
    ISBN 0-936197-41-2 (alk. paper)
    1. Headache—Alternative treatment. I. Title.
RC392.U73 2000
616.8'491—dc21   98-45868
                                            CIP

Natural Healing for Headaches
High-Powered Cures for Ending Pain

    Copyright © 2000 by Harbor Press, Inc.
    All rights reserved. No part of this book may be reproduced in any
    form by any means without permission in writing from the publisher.

Harbor Press and Harbor Health Series are registered trademarks of Harbor Press, Inc.

    Printed in the United States of America
    10 9 8 7 6 5 4 3 2 1

Harbor Press, Inc.
P.O. Box 1656
Gig Harbor, WA 98335

To my mother, Maria,

and to her healing hands. Her philosophy that any headache can be rubbed away by massaging the head with an upward motion has proved itself many, many times over the years. She has always found a willing and grateful recipient in me. A seeker of knowledge and answers to questions, she has always been an inspiration to me and probably has more to do with who and what I am today than she realizes. I love you, Mama.

CONTENTS

Foreword

Headaches can be a mystery, even to the most experienced physicians who treat them. Those who have most successfully pierced through the mystery and found effective solutions are actually the many patients who have gained knowledge and wisdom through their suffering. Dr. Urbaniak is one such patient who is in a unique position to guide headache sufferers on the path to healing. She is both patient and doctor, and thus is able to bring new insight and understanding to this painful and often debilitating condition.

As this important book explains, you can reverse a chronic headache condition and prevent years of suffering by simply making the association between headache symptoms and, for example, using sugarless gum or a certain brand of laundry soap, or discovering a sensitivity to chocolate or cheese. The remedy could be as simple as eliminating an offending substance from your diet or lifestyle, or using specific herbs or acupressure techniques.

A crucial aspect of Dr. Urbaniak's approach to healing—and perhaps the most important—is that she offers a variety of effective all-natural treatments, rather than taking the conventional route and promoting painkilling drugs that, over time, make the problem worse. Among the many natural treatment options Dr.

Urbaniak provides, you will find one that works for you. You will also gain a new understanding of natural medicine and the degree to which toxins, including painkillers and other drugs, permeate our world and threaten our health and well-being.

Although there are many possible causes and treatments for headache pain depending upon your own situation, there is a common path to healing—an increased awareness of your lifestyle and your emotional make-up, from the food you eat to the way you handle anger. Dr. Urbaniak expertly and with compassion guides you to this increased awareness by helping you to ask the critical questions that will ultimately lead to a solution for your headache pain.

Remember that there is an answer for everyone who suffers from headaches; read this book, and you'll discover what it is for you.

Fernando Vega, M.D.
Seattle, Washington

Introduction

It was September 1988, my first day in class at Bastyr University, and I had a migraine headache. The only way I could endure orientation was to sit near an open window and keep the classroom door open to create a cold draft that soothed the pain in my head. A fellow student, for whom the draft triggered coughing spells, kept closing the door. I would open it, she would close it. We went back and forth like this several times, until I realized I would just have to suffer through this one. I said to myself, "Well, at least I'm in the right place to learn how to get rid of this nagging pain!"

That was 10 years ago, and today, I am completely headache-free. What I focused on to heal myself of this increasingly common, yet extremely debilitating problem, was not a magic pain-relieving pill, but a look inside myself to see what could have been causing this painful situation.

The approach I used addressed lifestyle habits, such as avoiding alcohol (even minor amounts, which can trigger a headache); observing my diet and avoiding foods that seemed to be triggers; learning how to relax my body (not easy to do as one "jumps through the hoops" of higher education) through meditation, massage, and acupuncture; using the appropriate herbs to balance my body; and identifying and dealing appropriately with relationships that were causing unnecessary and unwanted stress in my life. Prioritizing also became a valuable tool in preventing headaches. Having too much on my mind or being overwhelmed with too many obligations caused headaches as well. This natural approach gave me permanent relief from headache pain.

I wrote this book because of my success using natural treatments to heal my own headaches, and my strong desire to help anyone who suffers from headaches discover what works for them. Through the wisdom of nature and natural cures, I offer you vital information to help you rid yourself of today's most irritating and sometimes most debilitating condition.

If you have ever experienced a nagging pain in the head, are plagued by recurring migraines or are a loved one of a headache sufferer, you will greatly benefit from this book. I present a holistic approach to healing, which is the only true path to permanent recovery. A holistic approach takes into consideration the entire person—the mental, emotional, and physical aspects of one's being—rather than just focusing on specific symptoms or problems.

If symptomatic relief of headache pain were the best treatment, do you think that we would need hundreds of over-the-counter medications and newer "improved" prescription drugs? Remember, the companies manufacturing these products hire expensive advertisers to convince you to buy their products.

Currently, there is a worldwide movement toward natural healing, the original medicine. People are tired of taking pills that don't work. That is why this book provides information that blends naturopathic approaches and solutions, including herbal relief, acupressure and massage techniques, dietary recommendations, and guidelines for taking supplements, and focuses on both physical and emotional factors—all in an easy-to-grasp format and style. I also discuss the inefficacy of drugs in treating headache pain, as well as the potential worsening of a headache treated by drugs. In addition, I will explain the important role of the liver in detoxifying drugs from the body.

Through all-natural means, I was able to cure my chronic headaches forever. In this book, I share with you my healing odyssey to help you choose the path that will end your headaches. My hope is that by reading and taking to heart what is written on these pages, you will experience freedom from unnecessary pain and maintain excellent health in today's fast-paced world. Remember, good health is normal; bad health is abnormal. Your body is always talking to you by using the language of symptoms to let you know if something is wrong. Listen to your body, and you will have a gold mine that will serve you for your entire life. Read on and discover the secrets of health and freedom from headache pain through naturopathic medicine.

CHAPTER 1

Anatomy of a Headache

Let's explore what causes headaches. First, it is important to determine what is actually hurting when you are having a headache, although this can sometimes be difficult. Some of the main causes of headache pain are:

- physical stress in the form of muscular tension and skeletal misalignments
- eye strain
- poor posture
- diet and lifestyle factors, such as irregular eating habits; food allergies; alcohol consumption; withdrawal from or excessive use of caffeine, nicotine, or other recreational drugs
- liver toxicity or congestion
- sinus problems, such as sinusitis and allergic rhinitis
- ear problems
- dental problems, such as temporomandibular joint dysfunction (TMJ; tenderness and locking of the jawbone joint), misaligned teeth, impacted wisdom teeth, and neuralgias (nerve irritation)
- organic brain disease or cranial diseases, which require a doctor's diagnosis or hospitalization for testing

• any problem occurring in the region of the head and neck, which can often feel magnified because it is closer to the sensory organs (eyes, ears, nose, mouth, brain)

It is also important to look at the emotional components of headache pain, for example, suppressed anger, or having too much on your mind. Although the source of such pain is psychological, not physical, the effects are just as real as if they were from a physical source because of hormonal secretions and changes that occur in many systems of the body when you are under this kind of stress.

In this chapter, we will look at the primary causes of general headache pain. Migraine headaches and cluster headaches will be discussed in Chapter 2. Always keep in mind that when treating any health problem, the whole person must be taken into consideration—mind, body, and spirit.

MUSCULAR TENSION

Muscular tension is a form of physical stress that can cause a stress or tension headache. In addition, the stress of daily life, work, family, and other pressures can rise above your ability to cope, resulting in headache pain. The stress or tension headache usually begins with a tightness of the shoulders, neck, or upper back. Most often, the pain begins in the neck and works its way up the back of the head into the forehead and temples. This type of headache is usually chronic and can occur at about the same time each day, most commonly late afternoon, or whenever you are experiencing an undue amount of stress. A tension headache can often trigger a migraine, so it is a good idea to recognize stress and tension early to prevent further complications.

In our modern world, muscular tension associated with the postural changes of computer work has become quite common. More and more people are using massage to avert this kind of mounting tension. You can use your 15-minute breaks most effectively by massaging your neck and shoulders to release muscular tension. (See Chapter 3 for specific techniques.) Some people are lucky enough to have a massage therapist available at work to massage their muscles. Ergonomically-sound office furnishings and proper posture also support the muscles and help prevent spasms and chronic pain.

Massage and other tension-relieving techniques will be most effective if you make an effort to improve your posture. For example, the typical shoulder slouch not only rounds the shoulders, but puts undue stress on the muscles and nerves of the neck and cervical spine. The muscles are attached to the bones of the spine and pull these bones out of alignment. This can be very painful and debilitating. Many people seek the help of a chiropractor when this happens. Chiropractic can certainly help in acute situations, but if your posture returns to its original pattern, the problem will return again and again.

Addressing the cause of the tension is the best way to cure the pain. When you walk and sit in front of your computer, check your posture to see if any improvements can be made. Simple exercises, such as shoulder shrugging and shoulder circles, can also be used to loosen your muscles. (See Chapter 4 for more on exercises.)

EYESTRAIN

Another common cause of headache pain is eyestrain, which is often the result of looking at a computer screen for long periods of time. Prolonged exposure to artificial light and the general eyestrain associated with computer work can trigger headaches. To prevent headaches caused by computer screens, make sure there is a source of natural light (a window) in each area where there is a computer, and take brief breaks by looking away from the screen and into the natural light.

Eyestrain can also cause headaches if you are wearing glasses with an incorrect prescription or if you are not wearing glasses and need them. These problems can be monitored and corrected through regular check-ups.

AIR QUALITY

Breathing fresh air is essential for good health. One example of the harmful effects of poor air quality is a condition called "sick building syndrome." With this condition, workers become ill from breathing the recycled air of a sealed building full of synthetic fibers, fumes, and dust.

Because fresh air is so important for good health, it is used as an effective naturopathic remedy for headaches and other ailments. While this may sound strange—especially since truly fresh air is rare these days—it is nonetheless very important for your health. The old so-called "nature-cure" actually consisted of just that—nature. Traditionally, health spas and sanitariums were built in natural settings where the air is fresh and clean—at the seaside, in the mountains, or in the country. Fresh air, sunshine, bathing, detoxification therapies, and massage were all enjoyed in a healthy, wholesome environment. Breathing deeply outdoors can bring fresh new energy into an aching head. Try it and see!

DIET AND LIFESTYLE FACTORS

I cannot emphasize enough the importance of diet and lifestyle in ridding yourself of headaches. This rather broad category includes several common dietary and lifestyle problems that trigger headaches:

- Eating specific headache-triggering foods (see Chapter 2)

- Over-eating or under-eating

- Skipping meals

- Food allergies

- Taking any kind of drugs, including street drugs, prescriptions, over-the-counter medications, and even the more socially acceptable drugs, such as alcohol, caffeine, and nicotine. Although there is a certain amount of euphoria or cessation of pain associated with using or abusing any of these substances, there is invariably a rebound effect. The liver, your main organ of detoxification, becomes sluggish, congested, and cannot keep up with the demands placed upon it. This causes your colon to become sluggish and underactive, resulting in constipation. As a result, toxic waste material builds up in your body and puts pressure on nerve centers, the brain, and the spine, thereby causing violent headaches.

Withdrawal from drugs like caffeine, nicotine, and some over-the-counter drugs can cause severe headaches, but luckily, they are usually short-lived and well worth the temporary discomfort. It normally takes only 48 hours to clear the body of these substances.

Everyone knows the sick, dull pain of a "hunger headache," which you may get when you forget to eat, but goes away after you eat. This type of headache results from hypoglycemia, or low blood sugar. Your brain thrives on just one substance, glucose, and if it doesn't get what it needs, you literally could be experiencing a "brain-ache." Proper nutrition and eating regularly is essential for good health and preventing headaches.

Dietary Recommendations

It has been my experience observing patients that we are all unique individuals with specific nutritional needs. To claim that any one diet is the best to follow could be setting you up for failure. But one very important dietary rule that applies to everyone and will help you avoid headaches, as well as other health problems, is: Avoid processed, packaged foods. They are usually laden with hidden sugar, salt, additives, chemicals, and colorants, none of which are good for you. Read the labels on all packaged foods.

There are a few sensible dietary plans that have been helpful to my patients seeking a more balanced diet. Some are new, while others have been around for a long time. Those I recommend are:

- Eat a diet rich in whole foods, which means eating foods that are as close as possible to how nature has prepared them for us. Purchase organically-grown foods without hormones or pesticides. Eat your fruits raw, not canned or frozen, and eliminate, or limit to special occasions, pastries made from fruits or vegetables, such as pumpkin pie for Thanksgiving. Eat your vegetables raw or lightly steamed or sautéed, and include organically-grown eggs, meats, and fresh fish in your diet. (Vegetarians use appropriate bean and grain combinations or prepared soy products, such as miso, to ensure adequate protein intake.) Make sure you eat a piece of raw food, fruit, or vegetable at every meal.

- Eat for your particular blood type. See *Eating Right for Your Type*, by Peter D'Adamo, N.D., to find out more about this eating plan. In addition to helping you eliminate your headaches, it can help you avoid chronic degenerative conditions.

- Eat according to your body type and the particular way your glands function. Read *Dr. Abravanel's Body Type Diet and Lifetime Nutrition Plan*, by Elliot Abravanel, M.D., for a very effective way to eat healthfully, drop excess pounds, and feel great. Dr. Abravanel's system of weight loss and body balancing is based on identifying and working with food cravings, and establishing a diet that will lessen or eliminate these cravings. For example, you might crave sweet (the thyroid or "T"-type) or salty (the adrenal or "A"-type) foods, and eliminating these cravings will put your body into proper balance. This will get rid of excess weight and relieve the stress placed on certain glands.

- Find out what your body/personality type is according to Ayurveda, the ancient form of natural medicine practiced in India for thousands of years, and use this information to steer yourself in the direction of correct eating habits. Dr. Vasant Lad's book, *Ayurveda: The Science of Self-Healing*, is an easy-to-read guide that will help you determine your body and personality type.

Digestion and Headaches

Before we discuss specific foods and food-related substances that can trigger headache pain, let's consider how profound an impact your ability to digest food can have on your health.

Impaired digestion resulting from just one factor, like too little hydrochloric acid in your stomach, can cause a cascade of events culminating with a toxic headache. When food does not digest completely, it begins to ferment in the stomach, causing gas, bloating, and an uncomfortable feeling of fullness. Toxic substances build up in the small intestine, and the liver becomes stressed from having to deal with food that has not been properly digested. This leads to a toxic bowel. When the bowel doesn't function properly, candida (a type of fungus), tyramine (a migraine stimulator; see page 26), and a variety of unfriendly bacteria grow and proliferate in the colon, compounding the problem as time passes. Congestion and pressure result, and a headache occurs.

Popping over-the-counter pain medication is not the answer because it does not address the cause—in this case, hydrochloric acid deficiency. Do you see how important it is to identify and treat the cause of a problem and not to cover it up with drugs that just treat the symptoms?

Food Allergies and Headaches

The foods you eat every day can cause your headaches. In fact, although cluster and migraine headaches are considered of vascular origin because of the effect on the blood vessels of the head (see Chapter 2), the cause for the blood vessel spasms can be found in certain foods and how the body deals with them.

Food allergies fall into two categories. The first causes an immediate reaction, like hives, when you eat a specific food, such as seafood or strawberries. These reactions are called immunoglobulin E reactions (IgE), and they account for only five percent of allergic responses. (Immunoglobulin E is a class of antibodies concentrated in the lungs, skin, and cells of mucous membranes.)

The second, more common type of food allergy can produce symptoms up to 72 hours after eating an offending food. These responses are called delayed-onset, and involve immunoglobulin G antibodies (IgG; a special protein that defends the body against invasions by bacteria, fungi, and viruses). Symptoms can include:

• Headaches

- Gas, bloating, and a lack of energy after eating
- "Allergic shiners" or dark circles or bags under the eyes
- Mucus in the throat after eating that won't go away, causing you to clear your throat repeatedly
- Joint pain
- "Mind Fog" or inability to concentrate
- Mood swings, irritability, depression, panic attacks, and hyperactivity
- Weight gain, edema (water retention), or inability to lose weight in spite of food restriction

There are several ways to determine whether or not you have food allergies. One simple technique that you can do yourself is the elimination diet. It involves eliminating specific foods and substances from your diet for a minimum of two weeks to see if you get relief from any of your symptoms. You then reintroduce each one individually to see your reactions, waiting at least three to four days between each newly reintroduced food.

The 10 most common food allergens, and therefore the ones you should consider eliminating from your diet, then reintroducing, are:

- Eggs
- Cow's milk
- Wheat
- Corn
- Soy
- Sugar
- Yeast
- Food coloring
- Food additives/chemicals
- Alcohol

When you're on an elimination diet, have a high protein broth when you're hungry, because eliminating allergens from your diet can create a kind of "false hunger." Other non-allergenic foods to eat when you're on an elimination diet are iceberg lettuce (organic), lamb, rice, and pears. These four foods are considered the least allergenic of all foods.

For those of you who have suffered for a long time with allergies, and have experienced symptoms such as headaches, severe skin rashes, eczema, and joint pain, it may be difficult or impossible to conquer them on your own. Sometimes it may be necessary to seek the help of a professional. Avoiding an offending food is very difficult for people with food allergies, especially when going out to eat. It is embarrassing, limiting, and can take the fun out of the experience. You might want to consider seeing a qualified NAET (Nambudripad's Allergy Elimination Technique) practitioner. This therapy involves bringing the body back into balance with the offending substance. I used this technique successfully for my own allergies, and then became an NAET practitioner myself. I have seen miraculous changes in myself and my patients as a result of this therapy. It has freed many allergy sufferers from their restrictive diets and lives. I strongly recommend finding out more about it if you have headaches that you think might be triggered by severe food or other allergies.

For more information about NAET, contact:

Dr. Devi S. Nambudripad, D.C., L.Ac., Ph.D.
NARF (Nambudripad's Allergy Research Foundation)
Pain Clinic
6714 Beach Blvd.
Buena Park, CA 90621

Phone: 714-523-0800
Fax: 714-523-3068

Toxic Headaches

The toxic headache is a dull, chronic headache pain that doesn't seem to respond to any type of treatment. It is probably the most common type of headache experienced today. Those suffering from toxic headaches are usually using pain medications regularly with little or no results. Toxic headaches can result from exposure to poisons, drugs and alcohol, or toxic heavy metals, such as lead, mercury, cadmium, aluminum, or arsenic. They can also be caused by toxic by-products left in the digestive tract from incomplete or faulty digestion from food allergies, intolerances, or sensitivities. In addition, toxic headaches can be caused by certain organs that are not functioning properly.

According to Oriental medicine, there are four classifications of the toxic headache related to specific organs. The **stomach headache** is felt on the forehead and frontal bone of the head, with pressure and pain around the eyes. There can be accompanying stomach upset, nausea, bloating, and even vomiting. The **gallbladder headache** is felt mainly at the temples, on one or both sides of the head. There can be accompanying indigestion or nausea. The **liver headache** is felt at the top of the head, behind the eyes, and there can be visual disturbances, like floaters or double vision. The liver headache sufferer is sensitive to light and noise, can become easily angered, and can experience wild mood swings. This is similar to the migraine. **The bladder headache** is felt at the back of the neck, but can spread to the entire head. Like the liver headache, this is also similar to a vascular type of headache, and can be associated with muscle spasms of the back, neck, and shoulders, fullness in the lower part of the abdomen, knee pains, and arthritic pain in the soles of the feet.

Since the toxic headache is so common, detoxification is emphasized when treating anyone with headache pain. (See page 18 and Chapter 2 for more on detoxification.)

SINUS PROBLEMS AND HEADACHES

The sinus headache is also very common today because of the high incidence of allergies and infections. Millions of dollars are spent each year on over-the-counter sinus relief medications. Sinus headaches can be caused by bacterial infection, viral illness, allergies, or excess congestion. What allows an infection to take hold in the mucous membranes of the body is a build-up of phlegm, mucus, and acids. Although the whole body is involved in this process, the pain of a sinus headache is so intense because the sinuses are encased in thin bone with little space for expansion when they become inflamed, and the sinuses are so close to the eyes and brain.

A sinus headache can be dull, chronic, and feel most painful in the morning. The pain can be frontal, facial, or around or behind the eyes. Many factors can affect sinus pain. Lying down usually makes the pain worse because it can increase pressure. Stooping forward or making rapid movements of the head also increases pain. Sinus problems and their associated headaches can be a mere bother, or they can pose a serious health threat and can progress to a very dangerous point. One reason for this is that the sinuses are chambers or reservoirs, normally filled with air, but in the case of chronic infection, they contain mucus and the products of infection, such as pus, blood, and fluids. These substances become trapped in inflamed membranes and cause severe pressure and pain.

One patient of mine, Angela T., had not been to a physician for her chronic sinusitis and had been treating herself with over-the-counter pain medications. When she finally came to me, I referred her for tests, and it was found that her maxillary sinuses had all but disintegrated from the chronic bacterial infection, and the infection was working its way to her brain. She needed emergency surgery and massive doses of antibiotics to save her life.

Some of the symptoms of a sinus infection are:

- A bad taste in your mouth that seems to come from your sinuses
- Discharge from your nose that is thick, sticky, yellowish-green, and has a bad odor
- A long-standing condition that does not seem to get better over time

If you have any of these symptoms, please see a doctor so you can get medication for the infection. It is important to eliminate an infection first, and then you can implement natural methods to maintain the health of your sinuses.

Natural Sinus Remedies

One natural method for maintaining the health of your sinuses is circular fingertip massage to the nasal and sinus structures. (See Chapter 3 for more on massage techniques.) Alternating hot and cold packs are also helpful in getting the sinuses to drain. The general rule for alternating hot and cold therapy is to apply three minutes hot, then 30 seconds cold. Do this three times, always ending with cold.

Nasal irrigation with a saline solution is another effective technique for getting the sinuses to drain. You can do this with an east Indian device known as a netilota, or neti pot, which looks like a very small watering can. You simply dissolve half a teaspoon of sea salt and soda in warm purified water and fill the pot with it. Then hold your head over a sink and pour the water into one nostril and continue as it drains out the other nostril. It cleanses, drains, and purifies the nasal passages and sinuses, and is basically free besides the initial investment in the neti pot. Water, salt, and soda are usually on hand. Or, if you prefer the convenience of a prepared saline solution spray, there are many different brands on the market you can purchase. These natural products became readily available a few years ago when nasal sprays were shown to cause more problems than those for which they were used. They dried out the sinuses badly and caused rebound effects that "hooked" users into needing them all the time. This is another example of symptomatic relief not being the answer to a health problem.

One 50-year-old woman I know cured herself of sinus problems she had struggled with since childhood using a neti pot. I met her when I was visiting her aunt, an elderly patient of mine. When this woman found out I was a naturopath, she was compelled to tell me her story, assuming correctly that I would be interested. Since childhood, she had been on every kind of antibiotic, steroid spray, nasal spray, and decongestant pill until her own M.D. gave her a neti pot and instructions on how to use it. She ecstatically proclaimed that that was the end of her sinus problems. You can imagine how this changed the life of someone who had difficulty breathing for most of her years.

Herbal preparations are also effective in treating sinus infections. A close friend of mine called me on the phone one day, upset and frustrated that she had been on several rounds of antibiotics which had not helped her chronic sinus infection. She wanted to know which herbs would be good to try, so I recommended goldenseal, plus an herbal preparation containing a small amount of ephedra, steam inhalation with eucalyptus and camphor oil, and ginger and garlic to be used fresh in food preparation. I also advised her to increase her water intake and to add lemon to her water. This approach addresses the bacteria (goldenseal), the need to break up the obstructive mucus (essential oils and steam inhalation), and, at the same time, decreases the secretions (ephedra). The pungent nature of ginger and garlic keeps the sinuses open. (Garlic is a natural antibiotic and is good for every part of the body, while ginger is very cleansing.) Lemon adds vitamin C and acts as an antiseptic.

A few weeks later, my friend called to report that she had tried everything I recommended, and her sinus infection was gone.

HIGH BLOOD PRESSURE AND HEADACHES

One of the reasons hypertension or high blood pressure is called the "silent killer" is that you can have it and not know it. In fact, the frequent headaches associated with hypertension can be a potent warning sign of this condition. Taking pain medication for this type of headache not only masks a significant symptom, but it can also be dangerous. Pain from this kind of headache can be knife-like at the temples, or dull and at the back of the head, and dizziness can sometimes accompany it.

High blood pressure is becoming more common and can have a variety of causes, or it may have no apparent cause. Stress and anxiety, pressures of daily living, emotional problems, worry, and the condition of our world all contribute to a state of mind that manifests in your body as tension, tightness, constriction, nervousness, and lack of flexibility, which can raise your blood pressure. Hypertension can also be caused by a diet too rich in fats and carbohydrates, which causes fatty deposits in the walls of the arteries. Mineral deficiencies, food allergies, and water retention associated with a diet too high in salt can also cause hypertension.

The approach to treating hypertension varies according to

your individual needs, but a natural approach is always preferable to the use of mind-altering drugs like the popular Betablockers, which cause more problems and harmful side effects. You can lower your blood pressure naturally by reducing your intake of fats, carbohydrates, and salt. Some form of relaxation therapy, guided imagery, or bodywork, such as massage, can also be very helpful.

Whenever possible, check your blood pressure. Take advantage of the free measuring devices often found in drug stores. Normal blood pressure is 120/70. High blood pressure is diagnosed when pressure reaches 150-155/90-95.

HEADACHES AND THE MIND-BODY CONNECTION

Tanya B., a patient of mine who suffered from severe recurring migraines, gave in regularly when having disagreements with her husband in order to "keep the peace." Her headaches occurred around these events with her husband. The outward "peace" she thought she was maintaining was creating anxiety and inner turmoil because she was unable to express how she really felt. Sometimes, our upbringing or the communication styles we learn in our families do not coincide with that of our spouse. It is understandable that if one partner was raised to calmly discuss matters of importance and the other solved problems by taking over and "being in control," problems are bound to occur.

How you deal with emotional stress has a tremendous impact on your health, particularly in the case of headaches. If your tendency is to stuff your anger or suppress it, and you have recurring headaches, you may need to re-evaluate your patterns of behavior and how you deal with your emotions. Stress in the form of suppression of emotion can have very profound effects on your physiology. It can be the cause of a variety of symptoms, including debilitating migraines, tension headaches, and general feelings of malaise.

If you feel like you have lost control in a situation, there are some things you can do to help avert these feelings from taking over your physiology and causing problems like headaches:

1. Find a quiet place and write down how you feel, describing your problems as you see them. Think of some things that could change the situation and write them down. Then bring them up with the person involved at a neutral time, not in the midst of an argument.

2. Talk to a close friend.

3. Go for a walk.

4. Take a long bath and add some lavender or rosewood oil to the water.

5. Curl up with a good book and a cup of chamomile or peppermint tea.

These activities have a way of helping you to unwind and to sort things out without having to put a great deal of effort into it. It shouldn't be hard work to discharge stress. It simply involves getting to know yourself a little better and becoming your own best friend. Good stress management can help you on the road to freedom from stress-induced headache pain.

ORGANIC BRAIN DISEASES AND HEADACHES

Headaches can also be caused by conditions such as a brain tumor (which is rare), a concussion, or subdural hematoma (a solid swelling of clotted blood between the brain and the skull causing pressure and possible brain damage) as a result of head injuries. The pain associated with brain tumors usually comes on gradually over time and steadily worsens. Pain medication

17

usually does not help this type of pain, and there are associated visual disturbances, such as light sensitivity, partial or total loss of vision in one eye, or problems with peripheral vision. Head pain can also be caused by lesions or tumors of other parts of the head, such as the eyes, nose, ears, teeth, or throat. These causes of headache pain need to be ruled out by your doctor and the appropriate treatment implemented.

If severe pain or visual disturbances **occurring suddenly** accompany a headache, see your doctor, or go to your local hospital. This type of pain can indicate the occurrence of an aneurysm (a ballooning of a weakened blood vessel, prone to rupture—a life threatening situation). Pain can also be caused by irritation of the brain's sensory nerves, meningitis (inflammation of the meninges, or coverings of the brain or spinal cord), or vascular (circulatory) disturbances, as in the case of toxic states like infection or poisoning, hypertension, or migraine and cluster headaches. However, in the case of common headache pain, whether acute or chronic, you can usually identify the causes and treat your own pain without drugs or other medical intervention.

DETOXIFICATION:
AN ESSENTIAL ELEMENT IN HEADACHE TREATMENT

When dealing with any type of headache—migraines, cluster headaches, sinus headaches, allergic headaches, or stress headaches—detoxification should be an important part of your treatment. You must get rid of the toxins in your body before you can be permanently headache-free.

Your body can be compared to a well with stagnant water in it. If you try to cleanse the stagnant water with fresh water, the end product will be more stagnant water. But if you remove the stagnant water first and then add the fresh water, you will have a new well containing fresh water. This principle applies to the detoxification process. Until the body is free of toxins, it cannot respond effectively to treatment.

Detoxification affects the liver first, then the colon, and then the tissues of the body—always in that order. Your liver is your body's detoxifying organ. It has the ability to break down almost any toxic molecule and render it harmless. If you take sauna baths and other physical therapies to detoxify your tissues, it can help somewhat, but if your liver is toxic, your headaches will not go away and, in fact, could get worse. Giving yourself enemas or doing colonic therapy is also of great benefit because it cleanses the colon and indirectly has a detoxifying effect on the liver. However, the cleansing process must start with the primary organ, the liver, for it to be most effective. Because problems with the liver are commonly found in people with migraines, please see Chapter 2, Migraine and Cluster Headaches: Causes and Cures, for a more detailed discussion of the connection between your liver and headache pain. You will be reading about detoxification throughout this book since it is so critical to any treatment for headaches or any other health condition.

A FINAL NOTE

Based on my experience working with headache patients, I believe there are three major contributors to the development of all headaches, including migraines and cluster headaches:

1. Food allergies or dietary problems

2. Sluggish bowel function

3. Compromised liver function or liver congestion

If you address just these three aspects of your health, in addition to your emotional and psychological well-being, you'll dramatically reduce the number and intensity of your headaches.

The chart on the next page lists 12 of the main types and causes of headaches covered so far. The first seven listed (through cluster headaches) are reversible through natural treatments. The rest need the attention of your doctor (conventional, or allopathic), strong drugs, surgery, or a combination of all three.

I hope this overview of headaches has given you valuable basic information to help you identify areas in your life that could be contributing to your headaches. In the next chapter, we will explore more about migraines, cluster headaches, and toxicity as an important cause of chronic headaches.

MAIN TYPES AND CAUSES OF HEADACHES

HEADACHE TYPE/CAUSE	SYMPTOMS	ADDITIONAL INFORMATION
Muscle Tension Headache	Pain can be intermittent or constant and worsening; feeling of tightness or stiffness, made worse by stress	Muscles of neck and shoulders may be tight and tender
Toxic Headache From infection, heavy metal poisoning, drug overdose, or alcoholism	Moderate headache, generalized, constant and pulsating; history of exposure to toxic or other harmful substances	Testing necessary (hair, blood, urine analysis) to determine substance causing problem, or can be result of toxins produced by the body
Sinus Headache	Frontal headache; can be dull or severe, sometimes one-sided; can involve face, eyes; can have purulent (pus) discharge	Can be caused by infection, upper respiratory illness, or allergies (allergic rhinitis); painful swelling of nasal membranes
Hypertension Headache	Throbbing at side, back, or top of head; history of heart or kidney disease; dizziness	Elevated blood pressure, edema (swelling), and retinal changes
Psychogenic Headache Includes anxiety, mind-body issues	Vise-like pain, worse from emotional upset; constant pain with no physical cause	Moist palms, blood pressure may be elevated, reflexes may be hyperactive
Migraine Headache (Vascular Disturbances)	Throbbing headache beginning in and around the eye, nausea, vomiting; pre-headache symptoms of light flashes and mood changes	Sometimes begins as generalized headache and escalates; associated with food allergies, liver congestion, and bowel toxicity
"Cluster" Headache (Vascular Disturbances)	Severe, one-sided, involving temple, eye, face, and neck	Eye redness on side of headache, tenderness upon touching arteries of neck, swelling of face, tearing, periods of remission
Tuberculosis, Cancer, Chronic Meningitis, Syphilis	Dull to severe headache, fever, history of the disease	Confusion, delirium, or palsy
Tumors of the cranium, eyes, nose, ear, or oral cavity	Mild to severe headache, localized to the area, generalized, or both	Surgery necessary to remove lesion and pressure
Brain Tumor (Increased Intracranial Pressure)	Mild to severe headache, inability to speak, vomiting, visual changes	Paralysis, mental changes, visual field changes may occur MUST SEE DOCTOR/SURGEON
Trauma Subdural Hematoma (From blow to the head)	Same as symptoms of brain tumor, or loss of consciousness	HOSPITALIZATION necessary
Post-Traumatic	After blow or injury to the head, pain is localized to the site of the injury	Pain can vary in intensity, duration, and frequency, and can worsen from emotional upset

CHAPTER 2

Migraine and Cluster Headaches

The word migraine comes from a Greek word meaning "half head," because this type of headache often starts on one side of the head. Standard medical texts claim that the cause of migraines and cluster headaches, which are similar to migraines, is unknown. Current theories suggest genetic predisposition, vascular instability (unstable and abnormal tightening and relaxing of blood vessels, in this case, in and around the brain), abnormal platelet aggregation (spontaneous clustering of platelets, or colorless blood cells), and sympathetic nervous system abnormalities (inappropriate stimulation of the "fight or flight" response). Findings, however, have been inconsistent so we're still not sure what actually causes these types of headaches. The cause of migraine and cluster headaches probably involves certain stressors that stimulate the above abnormalities to occur.

What we do know about migraines is that the pre-headache symptoms such as flashes of light, irritability, visual defects, and sometimes numbness of parts of the face and head, are caused first by a constriction of the cerebral arteries. Then the arteries in the brain and scalp dilate, or expand, and you feel throbbing head pain.

When the blood vessels dilate, they put pressure on the surrounding nerves, causing even more agonizing pain. Pulsating pain can be felt on one side of the head or both. The migraine sufferer seeks quiet, isolation, and darkness, and often experiences nausea and vomiting. Sometimes the vomiting relieves the pain. Ice packs applied to the head and neck are sometimes successful in controlling pain, and sleep also seems to help. Attacks can last for hours or days. Migraines can strike at any age, but commonly occur from age 10 to 30, are found more often in women than men, and may stop as suddenly as they begin. It is estimated that about 10 percent of the population suffers from migraines.

In one study that followed 30 pairs of siblings in which one had migraines and the other did not, an interesting psychological picture emerged. It was found that the migraine sufferers, or migraineurs, were more sensitive, had fewer friends, received less encouragement from parents and felt less trust towards them. Although this is far from providing a profile of a migraineur, it does bring to light the issue of sensitivity to one's environment. In fact, the other siblings in the study, who had childhood experiences similar to the migraineurs, suffered from psychologically-influenced health problems like allergies and asthma. This suggests a considerable psychological component. Along with treating the physical symptoms of migraines, psychotherapy has been successful in reducing migraine attacks by as much as two-thirds. This strongly suggests a psycho-social-emotional component in migraines more significant than previously thought. Research continues on this painful and baffling condition, and with each new study, we learn more.

COMMON MIGRAINE TRIGGERS

The migraine headache is actually a powerful response from your body, letting you know that an "insult" of sorts has occurred. What does it take to cause such a constriction, then dilation, of cerebral arteries? It can be food, anger, some sort of shock, fatigue, overwork, muscular tension, and so on. As I described earlier, many events occur to create a migraine, but the most common causes are:

- Allergies or sensitivities to foods, substances, or chemicals
- Hormonal disturbances
- Blood sugar imbalances
- Digestive problems (liver and/or bowel toxicity)
- Emotional upset or letdown
- Muscular tension (structural problems with the head and neck)
- Overwork and/or lack of sleep

Foods and Substances Commonly Implicated in Migraines

Studies have shown that the following foods and substances induce migraine headaches in susceptible people:

Alcohol	Coffee
Apples	Corn
Bananas	Cow's milk
Beef	Eggs
Benzoic acid (Soda pop additive)	Fish
Cane sugar	Goat's milk
Carrots	Grapes
Cheese	Melons
Chicken	Monosodium Glutamate
Chocolate	Nuts

Onions	Soy
Oranges	Strawberries
Peaches	Tartrazine (food dye)
Peanuts	Tea
Pork	Tomatoes
Potatoes	Walnuts
Rice	Wheat
Rye	Yeast

Chocolate, cheese, and alcohol can trigger migraines because they contain substances called vasoactive amines, compounds that cause constriction (tightening or narrowing) of blood vessels. Tyramine and dopamine are two vasoactive amines present in many commonly eaten foods. People with migraines caused by dietary factors appear to be deficient in enzymes that normally break down these compounds. Red wine, for example, contains tyramine, which can trigger a migraine attack in a person who doesn't have enough of the enzymes needed to break down the tyramine. Some drugs used to treat depression (such as Nardil, Marplan, and Parnate) also interfere with the break down of tyramine. If you are taking antidepression medication and you have a history of migraines, avoid foods containing tyramine.

The following foods contain tyramine or other vasoactive amines:

Aged Cheeses	Broad Beans
Aged Meats	Cabbage
Alcohol	Canned Fish
Avocados	Chocolate
Bananas	Citrus Fruits

Eggplant

Orange Pulp

Pickled Herring

Pineapples

Potatoes

Raspberries

Red Plums

Red Wine

Salami

Sausage

Sour Cream

Soy Sauce

Spinach

Tomatoes

Yeast Extracts

You can see why taking a closer look at your diet can be valuable in getting to the root of your headaches. You may need a little help from a qualified professional to determine your food intolerances or allergies, but you can certainly take an active role in the process.

HORMONES AND MIGRAINES

Hormonal changes are often associated with migraines. This is mostly true of women, who naturally experience more changes in hormone levels at regular intervals than men do. Some women experience fewer and milder headaches when they are pregnant. Many women find that they experience migraines more when they are menstruating than at other times of the month, and sometimes the headaches disappear after menopause. Other women who do not have a history of migraines may start getting them when they take birth control pills. These women should consider stopping the pill because of the association between oral contraceptive use and cerebral thrombosis (blood clots in the brain).

The hormonal cause of migraines is usually an imbalance of the two main female hormones: estrogen and progesterone. In most cases, progesterone levels are deficient. This may be

---

DO-IT-YOURSELF EMERGENCY TREATMENT

FOR MIGRAINE OR CLUSTER HEADACHES

(If the headache has already begun and cannot be averted)

1. **Apply ice to the head, face, or neck as necessary.** This has a local pain relieving effect and can suppress histamine in the area treated.

2. **Apply heat to the feet.** If you are able to sit up, place your feet in a pan of hot water, maintaining ice application to the head and/or neck. If you cannot sit up and must seek darkness and quiet, listen to your body and lie down. You can use a heating pad between your feet in bed. This is an old hydrotherapeutic technique called the derivative effect. Putting heat on the feet pulls blood away from the congested area, thereby bringing relief.

3. **Massage the neck.** If there is anyone nearby who can help, gentle massage of the shoulder muscles, neck, and head can also help speed return to normal functioning. (It is difficult, but not impossible, to massage oneself, especially when in pain.)

4. **Follow preventive measures.** Try to use stress management techniques, relax tense muscles, eat a healthful diet, drink plenty of water, and avoid alcohol and caffeine as these are important elements in bringing about long term relief of headache pain.

---

because our environment is so saturated with estrogen-like substances (such as pesticides and chemicals), and so much of our food supply has been tainted with estrogen. Estrogen is fed to cows to make them bigger and produce more milk, therefore, all of our dairy products—milk, yogurt, cheese, ice cream—are laden with this hormone. Progesterone supplementation is actually just a "band-aid therapy," because the source of the problem is our food supply. It is best to look for food labels that say **No Hormones.**

OVERVIEW OF MIGRAINE INSTIGATORS

The more common causes of migraines are:

- Foods, such as cheese and chocolate
- Alcohol, especially red wine
- Food additives, such as MSG and nitrites
- Hormonal changes
- Blood sugar fluctuations
- Fatigue (overwork/lack of sleep)
- Digestive problems
- Liver congestion
- Constipation/toxic colon
- Emotional upset/letdown
- Withdrawal from drugs
- Sun exposure or glare
- Muscular/skeletal tension

As you can see, some of the factors that cause general headache pain are also implicated in migraines. Also remember, as we discussed, there is a very strong mind-body connection when it comes to headaches.

Any of the above instigators, such as lack of sleep, overwork, or emotional upset, can cause hormonal changes, muscular or skeletal changes, or digestive difficulty. This illustrates the important fact that migraines are caused by a combination of factors. All of the contributing factors, or stressors, are significant, but it is the reaction to these stressors that actually brings on the headache. The best approach to curing migraines is to try to reduce these reactions, since they are really the cause of your headaches.

THE CLUSTER HEADACHE

The cluster headache is considered a type of migraine because dilation of the cerebral arteries is involved. However, it has been given the additional classification of histamine cephalgia. Histamine is a chemical substance produced in various cells in the body, commonly in response to allergy. (Antihistamines, like Benadryl, are used to block the release of histamine.) In people who suffer from cluster headaches, when a triggering event occurs like an emotional upset or ingestion of an allergen, the body cannot regulate itself properly, and histamine is released as a response. Histamine can easily cause dilation of the blood vessels, tearing of the eyes, congestion of the nose and sinuses, and a red, blotchy, swollen appearance to the face—all hallmark symptoms of the cluster headache. The clustering effect that occurs is peculiar to this type of headache pain.

The pain of a cluster headache is worse and more intense than that of a common migraine. It is sharp pain, usually at the temple or eye region on one side of the face. Then the pain may subside, only to return one hour later, or in a matter of minutes, again followed by a pain-free period, followed by more pain. Patients have told me they are awakened often at night by a piercing pain. They can experience profuse sweating, nausea, visual disturbances, numbness of the side of the face affected, and worst of all, a total inability to function. They cannot eat, sleep, think, or work, and have little choice but to stay in bed and suffer.

Unfortunately, at this point, many people resort to over-the-counter and/or prescription drugs. Over-the-counter pain medications and medicines prescribed by doctors, such as steroids, painkillers, and ergotamine drugs (used especially for migraines), all have side effects and many have the added danger of addiction. Pain-relieving drugs affect normal functioning at home, while driving, and at work. They dull the pain, but do not address the cause. You are then incapacitated by the drug, instead of the pain. Some drugs, such as codeine, cause a severe slowing down of digestion, which causes constipation, again compounding the problem.

YOUR LIVER AND CHRONIC HEADACHE PAIN

Another type of common headache pain is similar to a migraine, but given the general classification of chronic headache. Like the migraine, it is very much related to an overworked, congested liver, but usually has a slower onset or can be present in a low grade state at all times. Pain-relieving drugs do little to help the sufferer.

What exactly is the role of the liver in causing chronic headaches, as well as migraines, cluster headaches, and other types of headaches? Your liver has many functions that are critical to maintaining your overall good health. First, as discussed in Chapter 1, it is your body's detoxifying organ, and it has the ability to break down almost any toxic molecule and render it harmless. A healthy liver destroys histamine (see page 30), inactivates hormones when they are no longer needed, and detoxifies drugs, chemicals, poisons, and toxins from infections. Your liver is also a blood reservoir and a storage organ for vitamins, minerals, carbohydrates, and glycogen, which are released to regulate blood sugar levels. In addition, the liver manufactures enzymes, cholesterol, proteins, blood coagulation (clotting) factors, and bile. Bile is essential to the proper digestion of fats. It is an emulsifier, which acts like a detergent. Only half the amount of bile is produced by an unhealthy liver.

Research studies have shown that the standard American diet causes liver damage. We know that toxic substances injure the liver, and it is almost impossible to consume our foods without pesticides, additives, preservatives, nitrites, heavy metals from chemical fertilizers, and contaminated water, so probably everyone has liver damage to some extent.

Headaches are associated with mild liver injury. Some of the other symptoms are low energy, digestive problems, constipation, allergies, weight gain, and hormonal problems. A more seriously damaged liver is more vulnerable to inflammation, or hepatitis, which can be caused by viral or bacterial infection, or toxic buildup of chemicals, drugs, or pesticides. Toxic accumulation in the liver and the liver's subsequent failure to remove toxins from the blood may even cause mental disturbances. In fact, headaches, arthritis, allergies, anemia, diabetes, hypertension, obesity, alcoholism, and infertility all respond well to liver detoxification.

You can see that it is absolutely essential to look at liver function in the treatment of migraines and migraine-like headaches. Most allopathic doctors do not look at liver function when treating headaches because there is always a new and improved drug to inject, spray up one's nose, or swallow that is supposed to cure a migraine. Unfortunately, these drugs, which are toxins to the body, also need to be dealt with by the liver. Your diet and the use of specific herbal preparations to detoxify your liver and colon are your first line of defense. We will discuss these further in Chapters 5 and 6.

Remember that self-dosing with over-the-counter medications, especially on a regular basis, is dangerous and causes rebound headaches. The rebound headache is a sign that the body—the liver specifically—is no longer able to detoxify a particular substance, and as a consequence, this substance has built up to dangerous levels. Recently, Bristol-Myers Squibb created a new pain-relieving product called Excedrin Migraine. This product has been designated as a treatment for migraines, but if you read the label, you will see that it is identical to Extra

Strength Excedrin—same product, different label.

Through the "miracle of advertising," when the makers of Excedrin introduced Excedrin Migraine, doctors held a press conference to say, "Here, take this for your migraine." The doctors and Bristol-Myers Squibb apparently believe that migraine pain can be treated the same way as ordinary headache pain, but as anyone who suffers from migraines knows, that simply is not true. There is no magical ingredient, pill, or formula that eradicates migraine pain.

The danger of such advertising is that a person suffering from a migraine may be prone to take more than the recommended dose if the pain is not alleviated, thus activating the vicious cycle of pain and pills, and possibly risking dangerous toxicity from an overdose. Until the underlying cause of the migraine is found, any treatment, over-the-counter or stronger, is just masking the symptom of a problem deeper in the body. Many of my patients, at the time of their first visit, have reported continuous use of painkilling drugs for ten or more years. If the pills are supposed to kill or relieve the pain, why does it keep coming back?

A FINAL NOTE

The main causes of migraines and clusters have been outlined here for you. Look at your diet, your lifestyle, stress levels, and physical stress. Sometimes doing something simple like eliminating a particular food or beverage from your diet to which you may be allergic, can be effective in eliminating recurrent migraines.

Although many of the headaches we have covered so far may have similar causes, or one underlying cause, their differences are significant enough to warrant their distinct designations. And even though these headaches have many names, it is possible to treat them all using natural, effective, do-it-yourself techniques (except for headaches caused by tumors, or sinus headaches caused by infection that sometimes need to be treated with antibiotics).

The next four chapters in the book deal with some of these specific natural treatments. In the next chapter, you will learn simple acupressure and self-massage techniques that are very effective for headache pain.

CHAPTER 3

@

Acupressure and Self-Massage Techniques for Headache Pain

Acupressure is an effective technique for eliminating or reducing your headache pain naturally, without the use of drugs. The technique is based on acupuncture, but no needles are required. For acupressure, you simply apply pressure to acupuncture points with your fingertips. Among the many benefits of using acupressure and massage techniques is that, because they are totally natural, there is no danger of overdoses or side effects, and they can be done virtually anywhere, as often as needed.

Acupuncture has been used successfully in China and the rest of the world for thousands of years. It is especially effective in eliminating pain. In fact, major brain surgery has been performed with the patient wide awake using a few strategically placed acupuncture needles as the only form of anesthesia.

The acupuncture points that relieve headache pain run along nerve pathways, or meridians. When acupressure is applied to these points, headache pain is dramatically reduced or completely eliminated. Acupressure can be just as effective as acupuncture, and is much more easily administered, especially when you do it yourself!

When you apply pressure to a point that connects to a nerve, sometimes you may feel dull pain, a temporary "pins and needles" sensation, or an odd sensation of numbness. This pressure temporarily overloads the pain centers of your brain and prevents them from interpreting the headache pain signals clearly. In other words, the pain channels get short-circuited. What you experience, then, is the diminishing or elimination of the pain in your head.

Even though some of these access points are far away from your head (see pages that follow), they can block your headache pain effectively. Since pain messages travel through your complex nervous system, they can be intercepted at these points, where nerves come close to the surface of your skin and are within your reach. Acupressure works by sending impulses into these nerves, which are involved in a particular imbalance in your body. In this case, the imbalance is manifested as a headache.

THE GROUP ONE POINTS: FOR GENERAL HEADACHE PAIN

There are four pairs of easily accessible points on your body which, when pressed in just the right way, are able to access nerves related to headache pain. They are near the eyes, on the back of the neck, near the thumbs, and near the wrists. For simplicity, I will give them the names Head 1, Head 2, Hand 1, and Hand 2 and categorize them as the Group One points.

You may be surprised to find that you have already been using acupressure by intuitively pressing on points on your forehead when concentrating, or resting your head against your fingertips momentarily at work. First, let's find the points, and then I'll describe the specific techniques.

The Head 1 points govern the nerves of the face and eyes, and the nerves that innervate the muscles of the face and head.

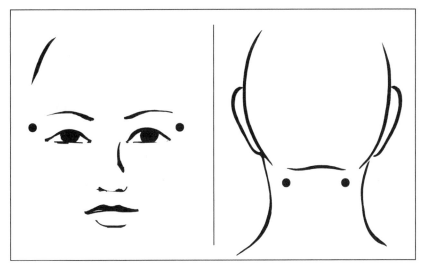

Head 1 Points   **Head 2 Points**

These points are at a spot halfway between the outer corner of your eye and the outer edge of your eyebrow, one finger's breadth back toward your ear from the bony ridge of your eye socket. The points are the small depressions just behind the eye sockets. If you go into the hollows of the temples, you have gone too far. You will know when you find the points because they will feel different and more tender than other areas you press on.

The Head 2 points govern the nerves of the back of the head, neck, and base of the skull. These points are on either side of the back of the neck, at the base of the skull. To find them, press on the bone behind your ears (the mastoid bone), and move toward your spine to the first depression you find between two large groups of muscles. Move your thumb in an upward motion, pressing against the skull and again, you will feel a difference when you are on the point. It will be more tender than the other points you press.

Hand 1 is considered a master point in acupressure and acupuncture. It is used for pain of any kind, and is located in

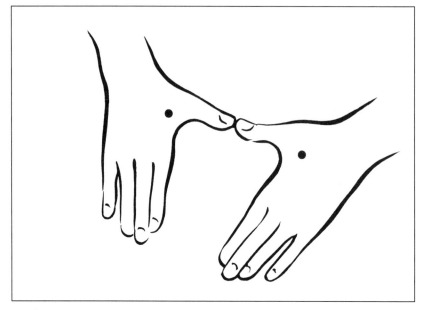

Hand 1 Points

the triangular area of the hand between the thumb and index finger. To find it, simply grab the triangular fleshy part of one hand between the thumb and the index finger, pinching it with the thumb and index finger of the other hand. Ideally, the thumb squeezes from the top of the hand, and the index finger squeezes from the surface of your palm. You will know when you find the point because it will definitely feel different and even painful momentarily.

Hand 2 points are found by extending and raising your thumb as far as it can go. Look at the one large tendon extending up into the wrist and a smaller tendon below it. The point is located in the depression between the two tendons, in an area sometimes called the "anatomical snuff-box," because people in past centuries placed snuff there and sniffed from it. You may press on the point with your thumb or index finger, but you want to press hard enough to create a sensation of pain or pressure spreading up into your arm or into your hand.

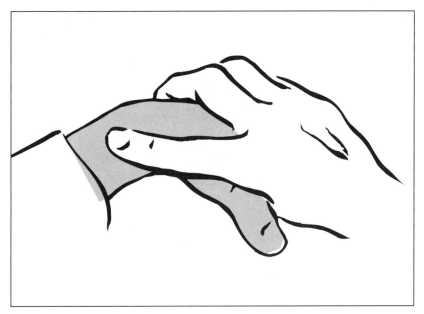

How to Find Hand 2 Points. Index finger can also press the point.

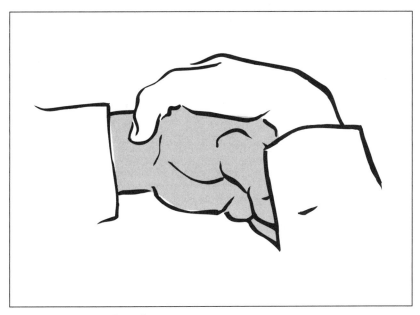

How to Press on Hand 2 Points

GENERAL DIRECTIONS FOR ACUPRESSURE

The following directions are geared toward acupressure techniques that you're administering to yourself. However, these general principles also apply if you're doing it for someone else.

- Although you may use either your thumbnail or index fingernail to deliver the pressure, if using your thumb, bend it so that the two joints form a right angle. This way the thumb can exert even more pressure. (Make sure your nails are not too long or sharp.)

- Press hard enough to make the point hurt, and hold it for 15 to 30 seconds, but no longer than 30 seconds per treatment. Compared to the pain you have suffered with your headaches, a short period of discomfort that will eliminate the bigger pain is tolerable and well worth it.

- Always press both points in any given pair. This is important even if your headache is one-sided. This gives a balanced treatment and prevents the headache from possibly moving to the other side of your head. (On hand points, of course, you cannot do them simultaneously so simply do one, then the other, in sequence.)

- You may use steady pressure or alternating (on and off) pressure, especially if the point you are working is particularly tender. You want to push hard, and push and ease off every one to two seconds for the duration of the 15-to 30-second holding period. You will find that the pain diminishes with each impulse, but do not decrease the pressure. Try to be consistent.

Applying Acupressure to Group One Points

> *Caution:* Do not use the hand points if you are pregnant. Acupressure is much safer than using painkilling drugs, but there has been suspicion in some medical quarters that it may contribute to miscarriage or complications with a pregnancy. Although the evidence to support this theory is only very slight and inconclusive, it is always best to be safe, and if there is even the slightest hint of danger, it is best to avoid the points. The head points, however, are perfectly safe for pregnant women.

When using acupressure with Group One points, follow these directions:

- Always use the four pairs of Group One points in this order: Hand 1, Hand 2, Head 1, and Head 2.

- Always start with the Hand 1 point. This is such a powerful point that it alone could banish a headache. Begin by pressing, using the previously described pinching action in the fleshy part of the hand between the thumb and index finger, using your thumbnail on one hand for 30 seconds, then the other.

- Next, move to the Hand 2 point. There are two equally efficient ways to access this point. One is to place your thumbnail in the "anatomical snuffbox" (see page 39) and grasp the heel of the hand being treated with the remaining fingers. This gives you added support in delivering the needed pressure to the point. Or you can lock the triangular fleshy part of the hand being treated between the thumb and index finger, with the corresponding fleshy part of the other hand. The index finger of the hand being treated will usually land on the point. This technique may not be as accurate in finding the point because no two people's index fingers are the same length, but if in doubt, just keep pressing in the vicinity of the point until you find that distinct sensation of dull pain. Then you will know you are on the point.

• Now, move to the Head 1 point. When pressing on the Head 1 point, you may apply direct pressure with the tips of your index fingers, or interlock your fingers and rest your forehead on them. You will find that your thumbs are free and in position to apply the pressure.

• For Head 2, there are also two equally effective ways to deliver the treatment. Use whichever technique is your personal preference. You can simply hold the back of your head with your open palms, pressing on Head 2 with your thumbs using a firm, inward and upward, hook-like pressure, lifting up under the base of the skull. Or you may interlock your fingers behind your head using the same motion with the thumbs.

You will find that as you work the points, they may get less and less tender. You will also see a marked reduction or elimination of your headache pain.

A fascinating aspect of auto-acupressure is the awareness that it brings to you and your body. Head 2 points, for example, are usually very tender when touched for the first time. You may notice how tense you are when you begin and how much easier it is to relax as you work the points. This awareness of your own body and the power this awareness gives you to take charge of your own health are some of the long-term benefits of self-treatment. It leads to learning more about yourself and what keeps you healthy and free from pain, an increase in overall well-being, and empowerment that you can do something for yourself that has lasting positive effects.

THE GROUP TWO POINTS: FOR RELIEVING SINUS CONGESTION AND PAIN

There are five specific points utilized for relief of sinus pressure and pain. Again, for simplicity, we will name the pairs Sinus 1 and Sinus 2, and the central point between the eyes Nose 1. These points govern the frontal (forehead), ethmoid (nasal cavity), sphenoid (deeper in the face), and maxillary (above the upper teeth) sinuses, as well as the nose and its nasal passages. Pain from these sinuses may be felt as eye pain, migraine-like headaches, and toothaches, respectively.

The nerves affected by the Sinus 1 points are the supraorbital of the eye and other nerves of the face and head. These points are located directly above the pupils of the eyes when looking straight ahead on the ridge of the eyebrows. Be sure to find the exact spot by noting the tenderness. Pressure on these points should be strong and directed straight inward.

The Sinus 2 points affect the infraorbital (governing below the eye) and maxillary (governing the upper teeth and cheek) nerves. These points are located on the top of your cheekbones, directly below the pupil of your eye when looking straight ahead. You may apply pressure against the bony ridge with the index fingernail, straight on, or with the thumbnail, with the fingers interlaced in front of the face, whichever feels better to you. The direction of pressure is inward and slightly downward. Do not press upward, or you will be pressing on your eyeball. Many of the nerves of the face are superficial and exit through holes in the bones and sutures of the face and skull. You will definitely know when you hit these points because you may feel a sensation of heat, numbness, tingling, or drainage, besides the usual dull pain when applying steady pressure.

The Nose 1 point is between the eyebrows. The thumb is

43

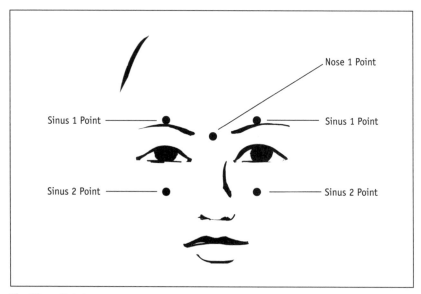

The Sinus Points

the best finger to use here. You can clasp your hands together and reinforce one thumb with the other for stability, or just stabilize one hand by supporting it with the other.

There is another point near the Nose 1 point that is effective for sinus pain. It is located on the flattened area of bone on either side of the inner edges of your eyebrows. This point will be tender like the others, but also has a sensation of traveling out from its center to the other parts of the nasal passages and face.

Inflammation of the nasal passages (allergic rhinitis) is often the cause of a headache related to a chronically stuffy nose. There is a simple massage technique taught to me by a Shiatsu master that can help relieve this irritating condition. Very simply, take your index fingertips, and starting at the top of your nose (between your eyes) massage either side of your entire nose, including the facial structures around it, with rapid, tiny, circular massaging motions. Usually relief is immediate; air passages open and drainage occurs.

Applying Pressure to Group Two Points

Use the same guidelines for pressure on Group Two points as you would use on Group One points (see box on page 40). Hold each point for 15 to 30 seconds. You will know you are on the correct point if it feels very tender. The Group Two points may need to be stimulated more often than those for regular headaches. Always press on the pair of points using these guidelines:

1. You may start with the Group One points, or go directly into the Group Two sinus points if you know your headache is a sinus headache.

2. Start with Sinus 1 points, then go to Sinus 2, and end with Nose 1. Again, if rhinitis is a problem, finish the acupressure treatment with the nasal massage described on page 44.

Utilizing the Group Two points effectively relieves pain, pressure, and stuffy or runny nose symptoms.

THE GROUP THREE POINTS: THE RECHARGING POINTS

There are three more pairs of points I would like you to learn about and use. These points are for recharging your mental, physical, and nervous energy. They are extremely simple to access and utilize, but the method of pressure and massage is slightly different from the other techniques described in this chapter.

The first pair of Group Three points, your mental recharging points, is located one inch directly above the eyebrows in line with the pupils when looking straight ahead. They will be more tender than other points, and can be found in the same way other points are found. The method for stimulating these points is to massage them using small, continuous circles, or in

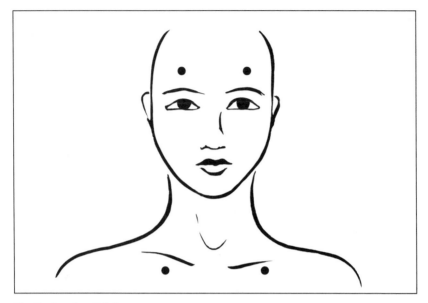

The Recharging Points

a back-and-forth motion.

The second pair of Group Three points is your physical recharging points. These points are located in the hollow below the clavicle (collarbone), directly in line with the mental recharging points. Again, the method for stimulating these points is to massage them using small, continuous circles, or in a back-and-forth motion. This can be done with the tips of the index fingers of each hand, or with the thumb and third finger of one hand, whichever is more comfortable for you.

The third set of Group Three points, which recharge the nervous system, is found in the soft tissue directly below the kneecaps. It is easier to access these points in the sitting position. Using the middle (third) fingers of each hand, simply place the pads of the fingers over these points. No massage is necessary, because this is an energy balancing technique. Just the presence of the third finger over the point gives plenty of energy to reprogram the circuitry of the nervous system. These points help bring balance back to an overtaxed nervous system.

To feel an immediate increase in your energy level, massage or hold each pair of Group Three points, mental, physical, and nervous system, starting with the mental points first. Massage or hold for 15 to 30 seconds, and you should feel your energy level increase significantly.

SELF-MASSAGE TECHNIQUES FOR RELIEVING HEADACHES

I'm sure many of you instinctively grasp at your temples when the throbbing pain of a headache occurs. Your intuition sometimes unconsciously guides you to effective pain-relieving techniques that you can administer to yourself. This is especially true for the tension headache. The small muscles of the face, scalp, head, and neck go through quite a bit of stress in the course of one day. Of course, it is wonderful to be able to go to a massage therapist, but if you cannot do so for whatever reason, or your budget or insurance coverage does not include such pampering, your hands can become great tools of healing if you just use them in the right ways.

First of all, if you have experienced anger, it is very important to remove its lingering effects. Remember when we spoke of stressors that can stimulate headache pain? Anger is certainly one emotion for which this is true. Not being able to express anger is even more damaging. An energetic cleansing massage technique that is very effective for getting rid of this type of headache is to "pet" yourself on the head. Start from the forehead and stroke your entire head towards the back, as if you were petting a cat's fur, lifting your hand up and away at the base of the neck. Do the same from the sides of your forehead until your entire head has been covered. You may use both hands, if you wish. Even if you have not been angry, this is a good way to start your self-massage.

The following list gives you other suggestions and instructions for eliminating or preventing headache pain using self-massage techniques:

1. Brush your hair and scalp vigorously from front to back to stimulate circulation.

2. Pull your hair in even segments with steady pressure all over your head. (This technique can actually free skull bone sutures that have become wedged together.)

3. Gently massage the hollows of your temples in small outward circular motions.

4. With the fingertips of all your fingers, massage your scalp through your hair, beginning at the temporal bones (above the ears) with small circular motions. First, travel to the top of your head, and always return to the temporal bones. Then go to the back of your head until you have covered your entire head. Pay special attention to areas that seem sore or more tender than the others, using the small circular motions. After giving yourself this treatment, your head will be tingling and you should already be starting to feel relief.

5. Reach around to the back of your neck with one hand and then the other. Bend your thumb, and with your opposing fingers, grasp the opposing group of neck muscles. Apply pressure with your thumb to one side of your neck, and deliver a kneading motion with your fingertips to the other. This area will invariably be a sore spot, but work the muscles with a kneading motion until the tenderness begins to subside. Your neck or head may get warm and start to itch a little at this point; this is normal. It is a sign that circulation is being stimulated to the stressed areas.

6. Reach up to the areas between your neck and your shoul-

ders, with your fingertips pointing back to the tops of your shoulders. You will find knots and tension in this area, painful trigger points that, when pressed, may send shooting pains up and over your head. Just rub these muscles forward and backward with your fingertips, moving back and forth from the base of the neck out toward the shoulder, until you feel a lessening of the pain.

These six simple self-massage techniques can help you eliminate or prevent a variety of headaches and let go of unnecessary tension. With the trained use of your own two hands, you can eliminate pain and live a happier, more balanced life.

CHAPTER 4

Simple Head and Neck Exercises to Relieve Headaches

Headaches often accompany neck pain and stiffness, usually caused by weak, cramped, or strained neck muscles. Neck movement may be limited, usually more on one side than the other.

Neck pain can be due to any of the following:

- Sleeping on a pillow that is too high

- Poor posture

- Extended periods of time in "the thinker's pose" (resting your forehead or chin on your upright fist or arm)

- Any blow directly to the neck or any sudden movement that snaps or jerks the neck

As I mentioned earlier, meningitis, a life-threatening illness, causes a severe stiff neck, fever, and headache. If these three symptoms come together, see a doctor immediately.

Prevention is the key to dealing with neck pain and its associated headache pain. If your neck pain and stiffness is worse in the morning, you may need better sleeping support. You may need a new, firmer mattress or a special neck support pillow. An easy do-it-yourself neck support pillow can be made from a towel. Fold a medium-sized towel lengthwise into a four-inch wide pad. Wrap it around your neck and pin it for good support. If your neck pain is worse at the end of the day, examine your posture and body mechanics during your daily activities. Avoid supporting your head with your hand.

You can also help yourself with the following isometric exercises to strengthen and rehabilitate your neck:

1. Press your palms against your forehead and push, resisting motion. Hold for five seconds, then relax slowly. Do this exercise three times, rest, then do it another three times.

2. Place your hand against the side of your head. Try to bring your ear to your shoulder, resisting motion. Hold for five seconds, then relax slowly. Repeat on the opposite side. Do this exercise three times, rest, then do it another three times.

3. Cup both of your hands against the back of your head. Try to push your head back, resisting motion. Hold for five seconds, then relax slowly. Do this exercise three times, rest, then do it another three times.

4. Place your right hand against your right temple. Try to turn your chin to your right shoulder, resisting motion. Hold for five seconds, then relax slowly. Repeat on the opposite side. Do this exercise three times, rest, then do it another three times.

If you commute to work, you can implement some of these exercises in your car utilizing the headrest. If you are stopped in traffic, you can do any of the exercises that require pressure to be applied from the back of the head. To strengthen the muscles on the side of the neck, you may simply turn your head to one side and press against the headrest. Shoulder shrugging is also excellent for relieving tension and pain from the shoulders, neck, and head. Repetitions of at least 15 shoulder shrugs is best. Always remember: Never continue to do an exercise that increases your pain.

If your pain is due to muscle spasm, you may use a cold pack over the painful area for 15 minutes. If there is no swelling associated with the pain, heat application may also be helpful.

Before you begin specific exercises and stretches for the head and neck, here are a few general guidelines to follow:

• Learn to stretch by feeling. Some days you will be more limber than others, so you need to be in touch with your body and not push yourself too hard. Stretching should feel almost effortless.

• Stretching is what allows for flexibility of muscles and joints. Exercise without stretching can cause tightening of muscles, tendons, and joints, which can contribute to more pain. Always stretch before and after exercising.

• Always stretch slowly.

Here are some general head and neck relaxation exercises that are excellent for maintaining mobility, healthy muscle tone, and prevention of headaches associated with muscle weakness, tension, or spasm. They are easy to do and do not require a lot of planning or thought.

1. The first exercise is very simple. While standing or sitting up straight, slowly drop your head forward as far as it will freely go. Then raise it up and let it slowly fall all the way back. Pay particular attention to areas that "catch," any grinding or crackling sounds, or whether pain is present. Repeat six times. If there is pain, or if the grinding sounds

do not cease after doing this stretch, you may need to see a health professional to evaluate a possible misalignment of your cervical spine.

2. Turn your head to the right and then to the left, noticing if there is any impingement or difference in how this feels from one side to the other. If you feel a pulling sensation more on one side than the other, you probably have a muscle that is in spasm or is tight. Hold this position for a few extra seconds and you should feel a lessening of the tightness. Repeat six times.

3. Gently squeeze your shoulders together forward six times. You should feel a stretch in the muscles of the back of the neck.

4. Sit or stand erect with chin in and chest out. Hold for the count of five and relax. Repeat six times. This stretches the back of the neck and upper back.

5. Sit comfortably with your fingers interlaced behind your head. Slowly lean forward, allowing the weight of your arms to gently coax your head forward just enough to stretch the back of your neck. Then come back up. Do this six times. This exercise also stretches the muscles of the mid-back.

Remember that stretching maintains the tone of your muscles, and exercising strengthens and builds endurance. If you have weak neck muscles, the exercises will be of great benefit, and if your neck muscles are in knots, the stretching is essential if you want to see any improvement.

Becoming more aware of your neck and head is also helpful in maintaining the health of your muscles. If you bend over to pick up a pencil at work, take the opportunity to let your head just hang there for a moment, stretching the back of your neck and letting the weight of your head help with the stretching.

You can develop your own special exercises and stretches to help strengthen your muscles and relieve tension. I have given you these suggestions as a guide to use as a foundation for achieving greater flexibility and strength of your head and neck. By improving the overall health of your head and neck, you'll be able to greatly diminish or eliminate headache pain associated with weak, cramped, or strained neck muscles.

In the next chapter, you will learn about the powerful healing effects of herbs in relieving your headache pain.

CHAPTER 5

Powerful Healing Herbs for Headache Pain

Herbs can be of great benefit in the natural treatment of headaches. They not only relieve the symptom of pain, but they also have other powerful healing effects on the body. In contrast, most prescription and over-the-counter headache medications have harmful side effects. For example, some products contain drugs that cause drowsiness; others have large amounts of caffeine. Tampering with an already sensitive nervous system with strong drugs in large doses can cause serious repercussions in the form of rebound headaches, dependency, and worsening of the symptoms. In addition, acute liver failure has been associated with the use of acetaminophen, the active ingredient in Tylenol and other headache medications.

Herbs are also rich in minerals, especially trace minerals, which are lacking in our soil and most of our conventionally-grown foods. Without minerals, the vitamins we take cannot be utilized by the body.

Herbal preparations can vary in their potency, unlike most manufactured products, depending on how much sunlight a particular plant receives, how it is dried and stored, and how long after being harvested it is processed. Herbs can also be used in many forms. They can be taken internally in the form of teas, tinctures, capsules, and extracts, and they can be applied externally in the form of oils, salves, creams, emulsions, and ointments. When taking herbs internally, tea is the weakest form. In ascending order of potency, tea is followed by tinctures, dried herbal capsules, fluid extracts, freeze-dried herbal capsules, and solid extracts. Do not be misled, though, to think that stronger is better. Sometimes an herbal tea can have a much more profound effect than other herbal preparations because it is warming and has an aroma, which acts directly on the olfactory center of the brain. Its effect can be immediate, whereas a capsule may take hours to dissolve, get into the bloodstream, and take effect.

An herbal tea is called an **infusion**. It is prepared by pouring boiling water over the herb and letting it steep for several minutes before drinking. A **decoction**, which is stronger than an infusion, is a liquid made by boiling the roots, barks, or stems of herbs for several minutes to extract their properties. An example of a decoction is boiled fresh ginger root. The liquid decoction is still usually called tea, but the way you prepare it makes it different from an infusion.

A **tincture** is an alcohol extraction made from either fresh or dried herbs. A tincture can be taken directly from a dropper bottle, or it can be made into a tea by dispensing the liquid into a cup of hot water. Placing the tincture in the water evaporates the alcohol but leaves behind the active herbal properties.

Capsules of dried herb vary greatly in potency, but are still an easy and effective way to take an herb. **Freeze-dried herbs** retain much of the fresh plant's properties and potency. **Fluid extracts** are 5 to 10 times stronger than tinctures, and **solid extracts** are four times stronger than fluid extracts. You will also see standardized extracts on the shelves of your natural health pharmacies or health food stores. A standardized extract of, for example, milk thistle, states the content of the active constituents of the herb instead of the concentration of the extract.

In the last several decades, there has been a tremendous increase of interest in and use of plant medicines by the American population. One of the reasons for this may be growing dissatisfaction with traditional medicine and its primary emphasis on pharmaceutical drugs. We also share a new awareness of the world we live in, and our responsibility to preserve and protect it. The subject of botanical medicines and treatments is very broad, but since we are focused on alleviating headache pain, we will discuss herbs specific to that condition and related conditions.

THE HEALING PROPERTIES OF HERBS

Herbs used to treat headaches are grouped into a number of different categories, or classifications. They are:

- **Nervines,** which strengthen and tonify the nervous system. Nervines can relax (called relaxant nervines), stimulate (called stimulant nervines), or tone (called tonic nervines) the nervous system.
- **Sedatives,** which calm the nervous system, reducing stress and nervousness
- **Hypnotics,** which induce sleep
- **Analgesics or anodynes,** which reduce pain
- **Anti-inflammatories,** which reduce swelling
- **Anti-spasmodics,** which control spasms
- **Febrifuges,** which reduce fever
- **Bitters and hepatics,** which stimulate the liver and help relieve headaches caused by congestion of the liver and gallbladder

- **Carminatives**, which are used for headaches caused by digestive disturbances because of their volatile or essential oil content. These essential oils, extracted from plants, soothe and relax the digestive system. They are called volatile because they evaporate quickly.

- **Aromatics**, which are also herbs that contain volatile or essential oils, but have the added benefit of a strong aroma that has an immediate effect on the brain through the olfactory apparatus. Aromatics also have an impact on digestion and the psyche. For example, lavender added to a tea blend soothes and calms digestion, and added as an oil to the bath relaxes frazzled nerves.

Some herbs such as peppermint have more than one property. It is a carminative, an aromatic, a nervine, a febrifuge, and a mild stimulant. You can also use herbs therapeutically in the form of an oil, such as peppermint oil. If you apply a small amount of peppermint oil to your temples and forehead, it can eliminate stuffiness of the nose and relieve headache pain.

A patient of mine, Christine B., is a nurse at a local hospital where aromatherapy has become the preferred postsurgical treatment for headaches caused by anesthesia. Small tubular chambers containing cotton balls saturated with peppermint, lavender, or other essential oils are held under the recovering patient's nose. These essential oils have proven to be a very effective substitute for headache medication, especially since the very pain medications given for headache relief are often instigators of chronic and rebound headaches. There has been a marked decrease in patient requests for post-surgical medications since the aromatherapy program was begun.

Before using any herbal remedies, see a naturopathic doctor if you are already on medication, are pregnant, or have a chronic condition. Never try to substitute an herbal remedy for proper medical attention. Because occasionally some people can be allergic to certain herbs, it is always wise to try a small amount and wait a few days to see if you have a reaction. If you develop any unusual symptoms while using an herbal preparation, stop using it at once. If you suffer from hay fever or any other plant allergies, be especially careful using herbal preparations.

HERBS FOR HEADACHES

Because pain is perceived by your nervous system, one of the goals in treating headaches with herbs is to restore, sedate, and relax the nervous system. But it is also important to think beyond the physical symptom of the head pain. You must also consider your mental, emotional, and spiritual state, and how these aspects of your being might be affecting your physical condition. By doing this, you will probably discover the root cause of your headaches, and then you will be able to address it. This is the only way to permanently get rid of your headache pain. Many of the herbs described here will be effective in helping you deal with some of these non-physical factors, such as stress, that might be contributing to your headaches.

Herbs that are effective in treating headaches and are commonly prescribed by naturopathic physicians are:

- **Valerian Root** (*Valeriana officinalis*) Valerian can help relieve migraine and tension headaches, and is often used in combination with other herbs. For example, an excellent formula for a headache with insomnia would include equal parts of valerian, skullcap, and passionflower. Valerian is also effective for "racing mind," paranoia, mental fatigue, and pain relief. It is a relaxant-nervine, a sedative, calms the spirit, lowers blood pressure, relaxes muscles, and is an anti-spasmodic. It strengthens and soothes the nervous system. Valerian has a very strong and peculiar odor. Some cats are sensitive to the volatile oils in this herb and will behave strangely, as if on catnip, when near it.

Dosage: Dosage is dependent on need, but as a tea, take one to two teaspoons in a cup of boiling water infused for 10 to 15 minutes; drink before bedtime. As a tincture, take one or two dropperfuls per dose. Doses may be repeated every hour, if necessary, not exceeding 12 dropperfuls in 12 hours. In capsule form, an effective dose can range from 75 mg. to 375 mg., depending on whether the herb is mixed with other sedative herbs.

Toxicity: Toxicity may occur at high doses. Although valerian is considered a treatment for headaches and anxiety, if taken in excess, it may actually cause these symptoms.

• **Skullcap** (*Scutellaria laterifolia*) Skullcap is excellent for anxiety, PMS, stress, tension, hysteria, seizures, and twitches, and has the added property of restoring the nervous system in cases of depression or exhaustion. It is a very potent relaxant-nervine, and renews and restores the nervous system while soothing nervous tension. The part of the plant used is the aerial portion—the leaves, flowers, and stems. Skullcap is safe for children who suffer from irritability and restlessness. If you have a sensitivity to valerian root, which is rare, you can use skullcap as a substitute.

Dosage: As a tea, take one to two teaspoons in a cup of boiling water as often as needed. As a tincture, take one to two dropperfuls three times a day or as needed, and in capsule form, potencies range from 50 mg. to 375 mg. Skullcap is safe and has *no toxicity* related to its use.

• **Passionflower** (*Passiflora incarnata*) The passionflower herb grows as a vine and has the most unusual looking flowers. The parts used are the flowers, leaves, and stems of the vine. Some people mistakenly think that the name of this herb suggests that it stimulates passion, but it got its name from early Spanish explorers who came to the New World and were taken by its unusual appearance. They felt that the flower represented the Passion and Crucifixion of Christ—the fringed corona, the crown of thorns; the three central stigmas that receive the pollen, the nails that pierced Christ's hands and feet; the five stamens, his wounds; and the 10 sepals and petals, the Apostles, leaving out Peter, who denied Christ, and Judas, who betrayed him; and some saw the cross itself in the center of the flower. No other herb has such an interesting background and strange history associated with it.

Passionflower is a very effective sedative and anodyne, a mild anti-spasmodic, and a hypnotic. It has a reputation for being a sleep and dream inducer because it contains flavone glycosides, which have been shown to reduce the breakdown of serotonin, a neurotransmitter associated with bringing on and maintaining sleep. Passionflower has been used successfully in the treatment of the tremor symptoms of Parkinson's disease, seizure disorders, depression, and neuralgia (nerve pain), including post-shingle neuralgia. As I mentioned earlier, it is often found in combination with other herbs in natural sleep formulas.

Dosage: As a tea, take one teaspoon per cup of boiling water, and drink up to three times a day, preferably one hour before bed. As a tincture, it can be used liberally, up to four dropperfuls three times a day. In capsule form, potencies range from 50 mg. to 500 mg., and it can be taken according to need.

Toxicity: Passionflower can be toxic and should not be used during pregnancy. Do not exceed recommended dosages. Symptoms of an overdose include a lowering of heart rate, blood pressure, respiration rate, and temperature, and can lead to convulsions and motor paralysis.

• **Feverfew** (*Tanacetum parthenium*) If you suffer from migraines, you owe it to yourself to try this herb. This beautiful and fragrant ornamental plant may even be in your garden. The green leaves are feather-like in appearance, and the flowers resemble daisies. Crushing any part of this plant releases a potent aroma, but the parts used in healing preparations are the leaves. Feverfew is an anti-inflammatory, a digestive bitter, a relaxant, a vasodilator (opens and relaxes blood vessels), and a uterine stimulant. It also eases the pain of arthritic inflammation, neuralgia, painful periods, and can bring on delayed menstruation. Feverfew also contains compounds that suppress serotonin, which causes constriction of the blood vessels, and inflammatory substances in the body. As you recall, there is strong evidence that components of both inflammation and vasoconstriction are involved in migraines. Plants like feverfew that have bitter properties stimulate and support the health of the liver, and you may recall our brief discussion of the role the liver plays in the development of migraines, hormone headaches, toxic headaches, and so on. For feverfew to be fully effective in the treatment of migraines, it must be faithfully taken for a minimum of one month and may be tapered off as needed.

Dosage: You can eat the equivalent of one fresh leaf, one

to three times a day, but feverfew is best taken in freeze-dried or dried capsule form because it is too bitter to eat fresh or drink as a tea. I think it may take away headaches because if you just taste it, you very quickly forget about your headache! Luckily, bitters are as effective in capsule form as they are fresh or in tea or tincture. For treatment of migraines, take a minimum of 125 mg. twice a day, morning and evening. For maintenance, once your headaches are under control, take 25 mg. twice a day.

Toxicity: Feverfew should not be taken during pregnancy, because it is a uterine stimulant. Also, some people are sensitive to the fresh plant and can develop contact dermatitis from handling it. In addition, some brave souls actually do eat one fresh leaf one to three times a day, and there have been cases of irritation or ulcers developing in the mouth. When purchasing your herbal capsules, always check the label for potency or how many milligrams are contained in each capsule.

• **Hops** (*Humulus lupulus*) Yes, this is the same hops from which beer is made. Hops is very effective in the treatment of tension headaches, restlessness, and insomnia. It is a sedative, bitter, hypnotic, and relaxant to the nervous system. Hops also has properties similar to estrogen, and excess use can result in gynecomastia, or abnormal breast growth in males. Hops is a fast-acting herb and can induce sleep within 20 minutes. It is taken best as a tea before bed. Do not take hops if you are suffering from depression because it can make your depression worse.

Dosage: For tea, pour a cup of boiling water over one teaspoon of the dried flowers infused for 10 minutes; as a tincture, take up to four dropperfuls at bedtime. Amounts in capsules can range from 50 mg. to 350 mg. Milligrams will vary with each bottle, as hops is often blended into other formulas.

Toxicity: Hops can be toxic in higher doses. Symptoms of an overdose are sweating, excessive sleepiness, slowed heart rate, dilation of the pupils, and diarrhea. Those who harvest hops have also reported skin irritation from coming in contact with the cone-shaped flowers.

• **White Willow Bark** (*Salix alba*) White willow bark contains natural salicylates, giving it a chemical structure that is almost identical to that of aspirin, without the gastric upset and bleeding that aspirin causes. It is an anti-inflammatory, analgesic, and a fever reducer. It is effective by itself or in combination with other pain-relieving herbs. Because of its anti-inflammatory and pain-relieving qualities, it is an excellent herb for migraines and headaches in general. When you want only pain relief, without the added benefit of sleep induction or deep relaxation, white willow delivers. It can also relieve arthritic pain and inflammation. If arthritis is present in the cervical spine, headaches are common because of irritation of the nerves. White willow soothes the nerves, as well as acting on the pain. I find it wonderful and exciting that there are natural substitutes for man-made substances like aspirin, which has some serious side effects.

Dosage: As a tea or decoction, take one to two teaspoons of the bark in a cup of water brought to a boil and simmered for 10 minutes. Drink as needed, or for a more continuous effect, up to three times a day. You can take two to four dropperfuls of tincture up to four times a day.

Capsules of the herb will contain anywhere from 100 mg. to 300 mg., and it is often found in combination with other pain-relieving herbs such as wood betony and skullcap. White willow has no toxicity associated with it.

• **Wood Betony** (Stachys betonia) Wood betony is an excellent herb for tension and nervous headaches, anxiety, neuralgia, and restlessness combined with fatigue. It is a powerful sedative, a tonic-nervine, and a bitter. The aerial parts of the plant are used for herbal preparation—flowers, leaves, and stems. Wood betony nourishes and fortifies the central nervous system, as well as having a gentle relaxing and sedative effect. It is especially good for exhaustion associated with prolonged physical or emotional stress, or for headaches caused by hypertension.

Dosage: For tea, pour a cup of boiling water over one to two teaspoons of the dried herb and steep for 10 to 15 minutes. This tea can be drunk over the course of the day, up to three times a day. For a tincture, take two to six dropperfuls up to three times a day. Capsules are usually found in combination with other relaxing herbs, but the dosage range is from 10mg. to 400mg. There is no toxicity associated with the use of wood betony.

• **Linden Flower, also called Lime Blossom** (*Tilia species*) Linden flower is best taken as a tea, and is not only palatable, but is a very effective remedy for the treatment of nervous tension headaches and nervous tension in general, hypertension headaches, and migraines. It has the added benefit of clearing cholesterol build-up in the blood vessels and preventing its return. Lime blossom is a relaxant-nervine, an anti-spasmodic, a hypotensive (lowers blood pressure), a mild astringent (tonifies tissues), a diuretic (promotes urination), and a diaphoretic (promotes sweating) when taken at a higher dose.

Dosage: Pour a cup of boiling water over one teaspoon of the blossoms and steep for 10 minutes; for a diaphoretic effect, use two to three teaspoons. The tea should be drunk three times a day. For a tincture, take one to two dropperfuls three times a day.

• **Jamaican Dogwood** (*Piscidia erythrina*) Jamaican dogwood is effective in the treatment of disturbances of the central nervous system, migraines, neuralgia, ovarian and uterine pain, and insomnia when it is due to nervous tension. The bark of this West Indian plant is a powerful anodyne, sedative, and hypnotic. The Jamaican natives have used it historically as a stunning agent when catching fish. It is non-toxic for human use if the dosage guidelines are not exceeded. This is a very potent herb, so access may be somewhat limited for the average consumer, but if you ask your health food store supplier, it can be found. Although it is non-addictive, the potential for abuse is always present for someone who may have a problem with dependency.

Dosage: Prepare a tea made from one to two teaspoons of the bark brought to a boil in one cup of water and simmered for 10 minutes. Ideally, this tea should be drunk only when needed for pain, but it can also be used as a preventive measure for migraine headaches if the pre-headache signs appear, or if you are able to gauge when you may be getting one. The same applies for the tincture, but one to two dropperfuls can safely be taken up to three times a day.

Toxicity: Do not exceed the recommended dosage. An overdose of this herb causes reflexes and blood pressure to become greatly diminished, nausea, vomiting, and convulsions may occur, and death may ensue as a result of respiratory failure.

• **California Poppy** (*Eschscholzia californica*) The California poppy can be used for acute pain because of its morphine-like properties. Native Americans applied the white latex from the plant topically as a toothache remedy, and used the whole plant as a painkiller for headaches, and a sedative for insomnia and headaches. This plant, with its flaming orange-yellow flowers, contains alkaloids very similar to those of the opium poppy, although it is non-addictive and not as strong. It is an anti-spasmodic, analgesic, anodyne, sedative, and hypnotic. The aerial parts of the plant are used—flowers, leaves, and stems. The stems contain the white latex that is also used for healing. The California poppy is quite safe, even for children suffering from hyper-excitability and sleeplessness.

Dosage: For tea, pour a cup of boiling water over one to two teaspoons of the dried herb and let it steep for 10 minutes. One cup will promote a restful sleep with pain relief. For a tincture, use one to four dropperfuls at night.

• **Lemon Balm** (*Melissa officinalis*) Lemon balm has a wide variety of uses. A common herb found in gardens everywhere, lemon balm has shiny, waxy bright green leaves and a distinct lemony fragrance when the leaves are crushed. It is excellent for depression, anxiety, uncertainty, irregular heartbeat, hypertension, migraine headaches, insomnia, menstrual pain, and it has a balancing effect on an overactive thyroid gland. It is also good for headaches associated with gastric upset (nervous stomach). It is a sedative, a general nervine, anti-spasmodic, carminative, aromatic, anti-depressant, and it opens the smaller blood vessels of the extremities.

Dosage: For tea, pour one cup of boiling water over one to two teaspoons of dried herb or five or six fresh leaves, and steep in a covered cup for 10 to 15 minutes. Since there is no toxicity associated with this herb, you can drink this tea two or three times a day or more, or as needed for a lift. As a tincture, you can take from two to six dropperfuls per day. The essential oil of this plant can also be used as aromatherapy by dabbing it on at your temples or under your nose, or dropping some onto a light bulb or in hot water to fill the room with the aroma. Lemon balm has a profound effect through the olfactory center of the brain, so breathing the vapors of the essential oil has just as powerful an effect as taking it internally, but it is not as long lasting.

• **St. John's Wort** (*Hypericum perforatum*) With all the media attention this humble herb has been getting lately as an anti-depressant, you should know that its effects are much more far-reaching. I find it validating and encouraging that the scientific community is starting to take notice of natural substances that have been used successfully for centuries. Significant research has been done in the last 10 years on the effects of St. John's Wort in treating some of the symptoms associated with HIV infection. It is also effective for mild cases of depression, and it does not cause any of the multiple side effects that many anti-depressant drugs do. St. John's Wort should not be taken for serious clinical depression. If you or someone you know has taken this herb for depression and has not found any relief, see a doctor.

St. John's Wort has a restorative and renewing effect on almost every system of the body and is effective in treating generalized pain, anxiety, neuralgia, irritability, tension headaches, menopausal symptoms, sciatica, joint pain, fibromyalgia, rheumatic pain, nervous debility, and stress. This herb is closer to being a panacea for health problems than any other herb. It is a tonic-nervine, sedative, anti-inflammatory, astringent, and it promotes the healing of wounds. In addition to being taken internally, it can be used externally in the form of oil, lotion, or cream to help heal bruises, varicose veins, burns, and sunburn. The tea made from the aerial parts of this plant is quite tasty and is very effective.

Dosage: For tea, pour one cup of boiling water over one to two teaspoons of the dried herb and steep for 10 minutes. Drink three times a day. For symptoms of neuralgia, take one to four dropperfuls as a tincture immediately when you get the shooting pains associated with this condition, or take one to four dropperfuls three times a day to build a level in your blood that will prevent attacks. Externally, apply the oil or lotion to the affected area several times a day to promote healing.

Caution: Although there is no toxicity associated with the use of St. John's Wort, excessive use of the herb internally can cause sensitivity to sunlight and a propensity to sunburn.

• **Chamomile** (*Matricaria chamomilla*) Chamomile is another herb effective in the treatment of headaches associated with anxiety and digestive upset, but it also has literally hundreds of other uses. The flower tops are the parts of the plant used, and they contain volatile oils, which render this herb highly aromatic. Chamomile is a very effective relaxant-nervine that soothes and tones the nervous system. It is a carminative, a bitter (yet is possibly the only bitter that doesn't taste the part), an anti-spasmodic, anti-catarrhal (breaks up mucus), analgesic, antiseptic, anti-fungal, anti-inflammatory, and it promotes the healing of wounds. It is completely safe for use, especially with children, and helps with teething pain, restlessness, irritability, and insomnia. Chamomile relieves gas, colic, and even ulcers caused by anxiety. A tea solution can be used as a mouthwash for mouth ulcers and sores, a gargle for sore throats, an eye wash for red, irritated, and sore eyes, and can be added to the bath water to enhance relaxation and stress relief. It has a restorative and renewing effect on almost every system of the body and is effective in treating generalized pain, anxiety, neuralgia, irritability, tension headaches, menopausal symptoms, sciatica, joint pain, fibromyalgia, rheumatic pain, nervous debility, and stress. Inhaled, it will speed healing from sinusitis and nasal catarrh (mucus). Applied externally, it speeds wound healing and reduces swelling from inflammation. It can also help heal skin rashes such as eczema.

Dosage: Tea is a very effective way to take this herb, because inhalation of the vapors has an effect on the nervous system (as with lemon balm) and on any sinus problems. The tea should be made from a cup of boiling water poured over two teaspoons of the dried flowers and left to steep for 10 minutes. It is best drunk after meals for headaches accompanied by indigestion. A stronger infusion can be used for mouthwash, skin application, adding to your bath, or a hair rinse for blondes (it promotes highlights). Half a cup of the herb boiled with two quarts of water is strong enough for these purposes. As a tincture, take two to four dropperfuls up to three times a day, or as needed for specific complaints.

• **Ginger Root** (*Zingiber officinale*) This culinary herb has shown promise in the treatment of migraine headaches because of its ability to reduce nausea and vomiting, and to inhibit platelet aggregation (clustering of platelets, involved in clotting). Using ginger root can lower cholesterol, and it has a significant cleansing action on the liver. This may contribute to its effectiveness in helping to heal migraines by reducing the toxic load on the digestive system. Ginger is a warming herb, a circulatory stimulant, a potent anti-oxidant, a carminative, and it promotes sweating. It is easy to find at the grocery store, and you can make a palatable tea from the chopped root. Ginger root powder is often found in combination with other herbs in capsule formulas because it acts as a catalyst or carrier, helping the other herbs to act more quickly and efficiently. Both fresh and powdered ginger are effective.

Dosage: Ginger root tea can be steeped or boiled, depending on how strong you want it. For a mild tea, pour one cup of boiling water over one teaspoon of chopped fresh root and steep for 5 to 10 minutes. Drink this as needed. For tea made from dried or powdered root, add one and one-half to two teaspoons to a cup of water brought to a boil and simmered for 5 to 10 minutes. Drink as needed. You can also use ginger in your cooking. The tincture form of this herb is highly concentrated, so if you choose to use this form, you can dilute it in hot water and drink as a tea, or take two dropperfuls at a time, three times a day, but be sure not to exceed this dosage. Ginger root has no toxicity associated with it.

• **Cayenne Pepper** (*Capsicum frutescens or minimum*) Don't let this extremely spicy herb scare you. The fruit of this pepper plant is cleverly combined in many herbal formulas, and for good reason. It is similar to ginger root in that it also can speed the action of other herbs. Recently, two research studies showed cayenne to be effective in preventing and treating migraines by desensitizing nerve endings to painful stimuli. Taken internally or applied externally, it warms cold extremities. People with cold feet have been known to sprinkle this herb in their socks for speedy relief. It is a powerful heart and circulatory stimulant, a circulatory and digestive tonic, a carminative, an anti-inflammatory, has cholesterol lowering and blood thinning properties, and supports the immune system. Not everyone can use cayenne. Some people cannot tolerate the warm sensation that accompanies the ingestion of the herb, but if you suffer from migraines, you should try it.

Dosage: Depending on your tolerance for spiciness, take one-fourth to one-half teaspoon in one cup of boiling water and steep for 10 minutes. Then take one tablespoon of this liquid and mix with hot water as needed. Tincture of cayenne is very strong and should be used cautiously. Take one-fourth to one dropperful three times a day or as needed.

• **Blue Vervain** (*Verbena officinalis*) This herb, although not often mentioned, can bring rapid and long-lasting pain relief and restoration of energy to the nervous system. It is a tonic-nervine, a bitter, an aromatic, relaxant, sedative, anti-spasmodic, hepatic, diuretic, and it cleans the blood and promotes sweating. Blue vervain is an example of an herb that strengthens the nervous system while reducing tension and stress. It also makes you more able to cope with stress. Blue vervain restores equilibrium to an over-excitable, irritated, overactive nervous system and does so very gently, quickly, and effectively. It lifts depression of all kinds, especially depression that follows a debilitating illness like the flu, and it stimulates a feeling of contentment. It is known to eliminate headaches in general, but especially migraines. It stimulates the liver and gallbladder, and calms a nervous digestive system, relieving gas, bloating, and diarrhea.

Dosage: For tea, use one to three teaspoons of the dried herb infused with a cup of boiling water for 15 minutes. Drink three times a day. Take two to four dropperfuls of tincture three times a day. Capsules are another easy way to take this herb, either alone or in combination with other herbs. Potency will vary with different brands, but an average amount per capsule ranges from 200 mg. to 400 mg.

We have explored the use of 16 herbs, some more well known than others, but all chosen specifically to guide you toward what will best work for you. I have a great personal love for botanical medicine because it brings us closer to nature and its gifts. I believe there is a natural remedy for any and every illness that man can contrive. To make it easier for you to choose the right herb or formula for your specific needs, I have summarized the effects of each herb discussed in this chapter in the chart on page 77.

To get the greatest benefit from healing herbs, it usually makes sense to take the capsule form, because it is the easiest to use. In addition, in some instances, herbal components may not be water soluble; therefore, the capsule is preferred, unless the tea form is specifically recommended.

HERBS FOR THE LIVER

Since the proper functioning of your liver is essential for you to be headache-free, use these herbs specifically to maintain the health of this critical organ:

- **Milk Thistle Seed Extract** (*Silybum marianum*) Take 100 mg. of an 80% standardized extract, one capsule daily for mild liver support, and up to three or four daily for intensive liver protection.

- **Barberry Bark** (*Berberis vulgaris*) This herb corrects liver function, promotes bile secretion, and helps gallbladder function. It is bitter, so you might want to take it in a capsule form. The average potency of capsules is about 300 mg. of crude herb. Take one or two capsules per day. Avoid during pregnancy.

- **Goldenseal** (*Hydrastis canadensis*) Goldenseal is very cleansing to all tissues of the body, mucous membranes, and digestive tract, and it is a great remedy for liver cleansing. Take one capsule, three times a day. This herb causes muscular contractions, so avoid during pregnancy.

HERB	TYPE OF HEADACHE					
	General or toxic headaches	Migraine	Cluster	Sinus	Tension	Psychogenic
Blue Vervain	•	•			•	•
California Poppy	•	•		•	•	•
Cayenne Pepper	•	•	•	•	•	
Chamomile	•			•	•	•
Feverfew		•	•			
Ginger Root	•	•	•	•	•	•
Hops					•	•
Jamaican Dogwood	•	•	•	•	•	•
Lemon Balm	•	•	•		•	•
Linden Flowers	•	•	•	•	•	•
Passionflower	•				•	•
Skullcap	•	•	•		•	•
St. John's Wort	•	•	•	•	•	•
Valerian Root	•	•	•		•	•
White Willow Bark	•	•	•	•	•	•
Wood Betony	•	•	•	•	•	•

HOMEOPATHY FOR HEADACHE PAIN

Homeopathy is the administering of highly diluted substances which, if taken in larger amounts, would produce the same symptoms that you are experiencing. These substances stimulate the body's own defense system and bring it back into balance. Homeopathic remedies are prescribed according to your symptoms, and the quality and intensity of your pain.

Here are a few homeopathic remedies and guidelines on when to use them for treating headaches. You can find these remedies at most pharmacies.

- **Belladonna:** For a right-sided headache that begins suddenly and severely. Your face is dry and red, and the pain is of a throbbing, exploding nature. Pain is worse with movement or bending over, and there is sensitivity to noise and light.

- **Bryonia:** For a violent headache and bursting pain aggravated by movement. Pain is better with pressure. You may be inclined to lie on your painful side, be thirsty, and have dry lips and mouth.

- **Chamomilla:** For a bursting, severe headache. You may be sweating, inconsolable, and feel worse with warmth.

- **Gelsemium:** For a dull, hammering headache at the base of the skull, as if a tight band is around your head. Your head is sore to touch, you feel heaviness of your limbs and eyelids, and you have chills.

- **Iris versicolor:** A classic migraine remedy. For a severe headache that can start on either side of your head and move to the other. You experience nausea and vomiting.

You feel very weak and crave sleep, and feel better with cold applications.

- **Lachesis:** For a congestive, left-sided headache. Headache is worse from sleep or starts while sleeping. Worse from heat and pressure, but better with cold applications.

- **Natrum muriaticum:** A classic migraine remedy. For recurrent headaches that start in the morning and progressively worsen throughout the day. Pain is severe, as if your head is being squeezed or is about to burst. Cold applications help. You want to be left alone.

- **Nux vomica:** Best remedy for overindulgence of rich foods, caffeine, alcohol, or tobacco. You are chilly, and sensitive to drafts, noise, light, and odors. Pain is behind the eyes and piercing, and is alleviated by warmth.

- **Pulsatilla:** For a changeable headache with throbbing pain. You crave open air, feel better with cold, and feel worse with heat. You may be weepy and appreciate sympathy, and do not want to be left alone.

- **Sepia:** For a headache with nausea that is left-sided, and can extend from the left eye to the base of the skull. You feel better with sleep and loathe food.

Remember, homeopathy works to bring the body back into balance with no harsh side effects and is one of the most gentle forms of healing available.

A FINAL NOTE

Although herbs are not considered drugs, they have pharmacological effects on the body. They help the body heal itself by normalizing and stabilizing metabolic functions. Herbs work with the body's natural tendencies. Chemical drugs, on the other hand, interfere with body processes by attempting to force the body to function in ways that are not natural. However, just as taking too much aspirin, acetaminophen, or any other over-the-counter medication can potentially cause harm, or even death, herbs can also be dangerous if used in excess or imprudently. Always follow recommended guidelines when using herbs for healing.

In the next chapter, we will explore nutritional imbalances that cause headaches, and the nutrients that are most important for preventing and curing headache pain.

CHAPTER 6

Basic Nutrients for Treating and Preventing Headaches

Many headaches, especially when they are chronic, are due to nutritional imbalances in your body. Adequate intake of fundamental vitamins and minerals is essential to good health and remaining headache free. It is important to understand that even though you may have an excellent diet, it is impossible to get all the nutrients you need to function optimally in today's world from your food alone.

Many factors contribute to the need to supplement your diet, including an increasingly toxic environment, stress, and taking pharmaceutical preparations, which rob your body of vital nutrients. An example of this is taking the birth control pill, which causes vitamin B6 deficiency, an imbalance of the mineral copper, and altered hormonal states which can cause other nutritional deficiencies.

Many headache patients on whom I do hair analysis often show high levels of toxic metals, such as mercury, lead, aluminum, and cadmium. These toxic poisons actually bind to your cells, pushing out essential minerals like calcium and selenium, causing health problems such as toxic headaches, fatigue, poor immune function, and even cancer.

Another problem I see regularly in headache patients, as well as patients with other health problems, is high copper levels. Elevated copper levels can result from sources outside the body, like tap water from copper pipes and water supplies that are naturally high in elemental copper. Copper toxicity can also occur from exhausted adrenal glands (a commonplace condition in today's world), a zinc deficiency (also common because of soil depletion and lack of zinc supplementation), copper IUDs, birth control pills, and a diet high in copper (nuts, beans, avocado, organ meats, and oysters).

Migraine headaches are more common in copper-toxic people because copper stimulates the secretion of certain neurotransmitters in the body that can cause arterial spasms or irritation of the delicate structures in and around the brain.

It is vital to follow a nutritional balancing program that will detoxify dangerously high levels of minerals like copper and other heavy metals from the tissues of the body. You can replace them with beneficial minerals and build up your body's defenses.

We know that we can either build up or tear down our health by the diet we follow and the habits we allow ourselves to get accustomed to. If you follow the guidelines set forth in the previous chapters, you are on the right track. However, nutritional supplements are also necessary to speed up the process of regaining balance in your life and becoming headache-free.

BEFORE YOU BEGIN SUPPLEMENTING

You recall from Chapter 1 that there are major dietary and lifestyle factors that contribute to headaches, such as alcohol and caffeine intake, skipping meals, eating irregularly and/or poorly, eating disorders, emotional stress and suppression of anger, not drinking enough water, and so on. Even if you are supplementing with vitamins and minerals, nutritional imbalances can occur if there are problems with your diet or lifestyle. For example, a diet high in sugar can trigger migraines. High sugar intake stresses the body, uses up the B vitamins, and can also cause a hypoglycemic headache.

In addition to dietary and lifestyle factors, you might have a nutritional deficiency that is the result of another physical condition. For example, iron deficiency anemia can be caused by excessive menstrual bleeding. In this case, supplementation can treat the anemia, but it is necessary to go to the source of the problem, find out why the excessive bleeding is occurring, and correct it to make a cure permanent.

Before you begin taking supplements, it is best to get your diet and lifestyle on the right track and to address any physical conditions you might have to give your body a chance to recover and rebuild itself. Then supplementation will be most effective.

For therapeutic treatment of deficiencies or for achieving optimal results from supplementation, nutrients need to be taken in amounts that exceed the RDA, or recommended daily allowance for a vitamin or mineral. The RDA was originally established to prevent diseases caused by a deficiency of a particular vitamin or mineral such as beri-beri, which is caused by a deficiency of thiamin, or vitamin B1; scurvy, caused by a deficiency of vitamin C; and pellagra, caused by a deficiency of niacin, or vitamin B3, to name just a few. The RDA for most B-vitamins is approximately one to two mg. per day. In contrast, most of the "stress formula" B-complex supplements start at 100 mg. of each of the B vitamins. You can see that the RDA guidelines fall far short for the therapeutic treatment of deficiencies that are common today.

Some of the major nutrient deficiencies associated with headache pain are:

- Vitamin B1
- Niacin (B3)
- Iodine
- Vitamin E
- Vitamin C

- Vitamin B5
- Vitamin B6
- Potassium
- Iron
- Magnesium

THE IMPORTANCE OF B VITAMINS

To maintain good health, it is essential to have a rich intake of all vitamins, especially the B vitamins. B vitamins are water soluble, are found in all green leafy vegetables, meats, brewer's yeast, wheat germ, prunes and raisins, and other foods, but they are easily destroyed in the body by stress, either physical, mental, or emotional, coffee, tea, alcohol, excessive sugar, antibiotics, tobacco, laxatives, and drugs.

A poor diet, especially one low in the B vitamins, can cause many serious problems, including headaches. Nervousness, anxiety, depression, irritability, apathy, memory deficits, mania, delirium, fatigue, confusion, memory loss, hallucinations, insomnia, and delusions are all symptoms of various B vitamin deficiencies. Besides a high sugar or poor diet, other situations that deplete the body of vitamin B complex are pregnancy, stomach disorders, disease processes such as cancer and the use of cancer treatment drugs, tuberculosis and anti-T.B. drugs, the use of oral contraceptives, anti-epilepsy drugs, and again, stress. The B-complex vitamins are necessary for proper functioning of the nervous, gastrointestinal, and endocrine systems, carbohydrate metabolism, appetite stimulation, prevention of wasting in certain diseases, stimulation of the liver and gallbladder, and reduction of sugar content in diabetes.

Certain isolated B vitamins are used as treatment for particular types of headaches. For example, a high dosage of up to 500 mg. of niacin, or vitamin B3, is used in treating migraines because it dilates the blood vessels and calms the nerves. However, niacin causes redness, itching, and flushing of the skin, which although is relatively harmless, can give an unsuspecting person quite a scare. With prolonged use, it may also cause liver damage.

Vitamin B6 in a dosage range of 100 mg. to 150 mg. is used to treat the hormonal headaches of PMS and medication-induced headaches (from aspirin, the pill, painkillers, and other medications). But if B6 is taken in dosages higher than 150 mg. to 200 mg. daily for a prolonged period of time, adverse neurological symptoms can occur, such as numbness and tingling of the hands and feet.

It is vital to supplement with the entire B-complex series if you are taking higher doses of B3, B6, or any of the other B vitamins because if you supplement with higher doses of just one B vitamin, there is a danger of causing an imbalance in the body.

Since it is difficult to get all the nutrients you need from your diet alone, it makes sense to take a daily B-complex vitamin to ensure the proper functioning of all your body systems. By doing this, you are not only making sure you're getting enough of all the B vitamins, you are also preventing a new problem from developing if you decide to take additional B vitamins to treat your headaches naturally.

AVOIDING AN OVERDOSE OF SUPPLEMENTS

Overdosing on some supplements is a concern, especially the fat soluble vitamins such as A, D, and E because excess amounts are not naturally eliminated from the body. For example, many people have begun supplementing with vitamin A as an antioxidant to improve immune function, for healthier skin, and for other benefits, but large doses exceeding 50,000 IU, unless prescribed by a doctor for a specific reason, can cause toxicity symptoms, such as severe throbbing headaches, fatigue, hair loss, appetite and weight loss, nausea, vomiting, and dry, shedding skin. The same applies to vitamin D, which we naturally get from sunlight and is often combined with vitamin A. Over 25,000 IU is considered a toxic dose of vitamin D.

Vitamin E can cause an elevation in blood pressure if larger doses are taken when initially beginning supplementation. Start with 200 IU and gradually increase your dosage over time. Most supplements of vitamin E are at a dosage of anywhere from 200 to 1,200 IU, with the average being 400 IU. A toxic dose of vitamin E is anything above 4,000 IU.

Excessive vitamin C intake, above 5,000 mg. per dose, can cause loose stools, burning urination, and skin rashes, although it is recommended along with bioflavonoids to stabilize blood vessel functioning when treating migraines nutritionally.

Some minerals can also be toxic when taken in higher doses. We already discussed copper toxicity (see page 82), but copper in trace amounts is essential for proper functioning of the nervous system, bone and blood formation, and wound healing. The average dose of copper in mineral or vitamin supplements is 2 mg. to 3 mg. More than 40 mg. is considered a toxic dose. Selenium, a trace mineral which is very effective in removing toxic metals from the body, is usually found in dosages ranging from 50 mcg. to 250 mcg. Therapeutic dosages can go as high as 500 mcg. per day, depending on the need. Above 500 mg. is considered toxic and can cause jaundice, skin eruptions, and a strong garlic-like odor on the breath. Remember, there is quite a jump between micrograms (mcg.) and milligrams (mg.). There are 1,000 micrograms in one milligram, so you would have to take a thousand 500 mcg. tablets to reach toxicity.

Iron, which is particularly important to women's health, is one of the minerals you should not supplement with unless blood or other tests have shown a deficiency. It has an RDA of 18 mg. per day, but therapeutic doses to treat anemia can range as high as 50 mg. per day. Toxicity can occur at 100 mg.

Another mineral that has a known toxicity level is magnesium. Magnesium is used for treating a variety of conditions including migraine headaches and hypertension; the dosage ranges from 300 mg. to 1,000 mg. Even at therapeutic doses, magnesium can cause flushing due to arterial relaxation, and loose stools due to relaxation of the smooth muscle of the intestinal tract. Toxicity occurs at 30,000 mg. You can see that even substances that are considered safe and natural like vitamins can do harm if taken carelessly. The same applies to over-the-counter medications.

Many patients who have come to see me reporting recurrent chronic headaches regularly take a variety of over-the-counter and prescription medications like acetaminophen, aspirin, and steroidal and non-steroidal anti-inflammatories. Significant side effects may continue even with sporadic use. Aspirin causes gastrointestinal irritation, ulceration and bleeding, and prolonged bleeding time. Other NSAIDs (non-steroidal anti-inflammatory drugs), such as ibuprofen, naproxen, and indomethacin, also cause GI upset and bleeding, abdominal pain, diarrhea, nausea, increased chance of hepatitis, liver enzyme abnormalities, kidney toxicity, prolonged bleeding, and edema (swelling). Acetaminophen, the main ingredient in Tylenol, can be toxic to the liver and kidneys even in small amounts, depending on the health of the person taking it. Steroids cause the same stomach problems as these other drugs, but also edema, increased fat deposition, muscle wasting, shrinking of the adrenal glands, fatigue, low blood pressure, low tolerance to stress, osteoporosis, mood changes, insomnia, depression, irritability, poor wound healing, glaucoma, and cataracts. Some of the newer vasoconstrictor migraine headache medications like sumatriptan (Imitrex) help sufferers if taken immediately at the onset of symptoms, but the side effects are significant, and it is still just a quick fix—something to deal with the immediate symptom of a migraine (vasodilation and pain), not the cause.

In spite of the side effects from all of these medications, and the rebound headaches that can occur with many of them, people continue to use them almost as a conditioned response or out of fear of the pain. Effective natural treatment of headaches requires stopping the use of these drugs because they interfere with the body's own natural pain-relieving mechanisms. Drugs also deplete your body of essential nutrients, making it necessary for you to increase vitamin and mineral supplementation. Once you make a commitment to healing your headaches the natural way, you'll never need to take any more of these unnatural compounds.

TREATING YOUR HEADACHES WITH SUPPLEMENTS

Here is a supplement plan for treating and preventing all types of headaches. To treat migraines, you'll need increased amounts of magnesium, calcium, and potassium. See the box on page 89 for specific guidelines.

For women who experience migraines near or during their periods, calcium and magnesium may be increased for prevention as needed, up to acute dosages. Remember that diet is also important in avoiding migraines (see Chapters 1 and 2).

Here is a supplement plan for treating a migraine as soon as you feel it coming on:

FOR TREATING AND PREVENTING ALL HEADACHE PAIN			
Daily Maintenance			
Minerals	**Vitamins**	**Additional Information**	**Additional Support**
Calcium 500 mg.	B-Complex 50 mg.	Take vitamins with food	Fresh air, exercise
Magnesium 500 mg.	B6 50 mg.	Eat meats and grains in moderation	Plenty of rest
Potassium 100 mg.	Vitamin C with bioflavonoids 500-1000 mg.	Have smaller, more frequent meals	Fresh juices in season
	Vitamin B3 (niacin) 50 mg.	If flushing with B3 is uncomfortable, get niacinamide or other formulas that don't cause it	Drink more pure water
Selenium 50 mcg.	Vitamin E 200-1,000 IU according to needs	Selenium detoxifies heavy metals, is an anti-oxidant, and augments vitamin E activity	Deep breathing exercises
	Pantothenic acid (B5) 100 mg.	Anti-stress, increases vitality, protects nervous system	

FOR MIGRAINE HEADACHES, ACUTE PHASE			
(If you feel one coming on)			
MINERALS	**VITAMINS**	**ADDITIONAL INFORMATION**	**ADDITIONAL SUPPORT**
Magnesium 1000 mg.		Magnesium stabilizes and relaxes blood vessels, soothes nerves, and eliminates spasms, tremors and tension	Hot or cold compresses, whichever feels best. Lie down and rest until relief occurs.
Calcium 1000 mg		Eases anxiety, pain, muscular cramps and twitching, irritability and achiness.	Eat something bland—a piece of dark toast or a banana if taking supplements on an empty stomach.
Potassium 200 mg.		Normalizes nervous system and hormonal secretions, and prevents over-acidity.	

Regardless of the cause of the migraine, this emergency treatment should help you avert it or stop it altogether. Minerals help to maintain balance in the body, are catalysts in many enzyme reactions, and speed all healing processes. As you can see from the box on page 89, you also need to take vitamins to prevent migraines, but because in the acute phase of a migraine there is often nausea and vomiting, vitamins could aggravate the condition.

Additional Guidelines for Specific Types of Headaches

Here are treatment guidelines for specific types of headaches that include supplementation, as well as additional support:

- **General or Toxic Headaches:** In the case of general or toxic headaches, follow the vitamin and mineral guidelines on page 89, but also consider colon detoxification, cleansing teas, and additional liver cleansing. Colon detoxification

---

Cleansing Tea

Here is a recipe for cleansing tea.
Combine the herbs together, then take as a tea before going to bed.

Dandelion Root, two parts (liver detoxifier)

Dandelion leaf, one part (diuretic)

Yellow Dock, two parts (gentle laxative and detoxifier)

Senna, one part (purgative, laxative)

Licorice, one part (soothing to the digestive tract)

Ginger, one part (soothing and stimulating to liver and digestion)

These herbs can be purchased at most health food stores.

---

can be accomplished by starting on psyllium seed fiber (the main ingredient in Metamucil) drunk daily with lots of water, enemas of warm water or organic coffee (very detoxifying to the liver), and colonic irrigation provided by your naturopathic clinic. If slow or sluggish bowel function is a problem, it might be wise to begin with some cleansing teas to get things moving before you use bulking agents like psyllium seed. Some people report a worsening of constipation after they begin using bulking agents.

Since the proper functioning of the liver is critical to curing these and all types of headaches, you should also be taking herbs that are used specifically for maintaining the health of your liver. See Chapter 5 for recommendations.

• **Migraine Headaches:** Follow the recommendations in the charts, and pay close attention to diet and stressors that can trigger migraines. Using acupressure can also help in acute situations. See Chapter 3 for specific recommendations. In addition, use herbs that are especially effective in maintaining the health of your liver (see Chapter 5).

• **Cluster Headaches:** Follow the recommendations for migraines, but add 500 mg. daily of bioflavonoids, such as quercitin. Quercitin stabilizes mast cells which are involved in histamine release (see Chapter 2, page 30).

• **Sinus Headaches:** Take supplements as suggested in the chart on page 89, but include 15,000-25,000 IU of vitamin A and/or 25,000 to 50,000 IU of beta-carotene, and up to 5,000 mg. of vitamin C in divided doses over the course of the day for immune support. Hot compresses or alternating hot and cold applications can help drain and heal sinus passages. Also try inhalation therapy with oils of eucalyptus and camphor, which will break up mucus and infection. Inhalation therapy can be accomplished either by using steam or by direct inhalation of the oils held under the nose on a cotton ball. For steam inhalation, boil water in a two-to four-quart pot. Place a towel over your head and let it hang down around the steamy pot. Add three drops each of eucalyptus oil and camphor oil into the boiling water, and breathe as deeply as you can. Repeat as the oil dissipates. The great benefit of using steam is that the particles of oil actually join the steam molecules, and you are able to get the oil to penetrate deeper into the nasal and sinus structures.

• **Tension Headaches:** In addition to following all the guidelines presented here, avoid stimulants, consciously work on relaxing tight muscles, and seek peace and calm.

• **Psychogenic Headaches (Mind-Body):** Follow all guidelines, but be particularly aware of stress and suppressed emotions, specifically, anger. Get involved in some form of exercise that can help you "blow off steam."

Please be aware that although only a few vitamins and minerals are usually given specifically for any one condition, in every condition of poor or failing health, or even less than optimal health, it is wise to make sure you supplement with all the known vitamins and minerals, preferably natural versus synthetic. Many vitamins and minerals are available in organically-grown foods, sea kelp, brewer's yeast, and other sources.

I have given you guidelines here that will help you not only eliminate your headaches, but improve your overall health as well. Keep in mind, however, that you must take into consideration your own individual biochemistry and personality to get to the bottom of what is causing your headaches. Each person is unique and has individual needs. You may need to do some soul searching or reevaluating of your life to decide which changes you are going to make to treat your headaches most effectively.

A Final Word

I hope that the information presented here has been useful to you and your loved ones. It would be wonderful if we never got sick or experienced pain. But often, pain can be an opportunity to learn something about ourselves.

It is easy to take health for granted while you're healthy. Healing from pain and illness is something your body unconsciously strives to do 24 hours a day. This process is as neverending as your breathing or heartbeat. When your body does not heal itself, it means that something is getting in the way of its innate ability to heal. The goal is always to remove any obstacles to cure, and to give your body what it needs to allow it to do the work it was programmed to do.

My journey in healing my own migraine headaches caused me to look at where I was out of balance, where I was not listening to the language of my body, and where I was pushing myself without taking a break. I hope that sharing what I've learned from my journey will make yours easier.

As with healing from any condition, you need to change the circumstances that brought about the malfunction in the first place. Remember that pain is a protest from your body that it is being subjected to some form of abuse. What's causing the pain comes from the conditions under which you are requiring your body to function. Most of the time, we don't know what we did wrong to make us sick. It has been my intention in this book to give you an understanding of how your diet, lifestyle habits, and emotions affect your physiology and, ultimately, your health. Gaining control over your health requires gaining control over your life and making choices that benefit you. Your body was designed to last a long time. That span can be cut short if you don't follow the natural laws that govern us all. The door is always open to those who seek to journey back to wellness. You just have to take that first step.

REFERENCES

Airola, Paavo. *How to Get Well.* Phoenix, AZ: Health Plus Publishers, 1974.

Blacklow, R.S. *MacBrydes Signs and Symptoms,* Sixth Edition. New York: J.B. Lippincott, 1983.

Davis, Adelle. *Let's Get Well.* New York: Harcourt, Brace, Jovanovich, 1965.

Girdano, Daniel, and George Everly. *Controlling Stress and Tension—A Holistic Approach.* Englewood Cliffs, NJ: Prentice Hall, 1979.

Grant, E.C.G. Food Allergies and Migraine. *Lancet* i: 966-9, 1979.

Hoffmann, David. *The Holistic Herbal,* Third Edition. Longmead, Shaftesbury, Dorset, England: Element Books Ltd., 1988.

Hoffman, David. *The Herb User's Guide.* Wellingborough, Northhamptonshire, England: Thorsons Publishers Ltd., 1987.

Isler, H. *Advances in Migraine Research and Therapy.* New York: Raven Press, 1982.

Krause, Marie V. and L. Kathleen Mahan. *Food, Nutrition, and Diet Therapy,* Seventh Edition. Philadelphia: W.B. Saunders Company, 1984.

Kurland, Howard D. *Quick Headache Relief Without Drugs.* New York: Ballantine Books, 1977.

Michaud, Ellen, Lila L. Anastas, and editors of *Prevention Magazine. Listen to Your Body.* Emmaus, PA: Rodale Press, 1988.

Murray, Michael and Joseph Pizzorno. *Encyclopedia of Natural Medicine.* Rocklin, CA: Prima Publishing, 1990.

Murray, Michael. Migraine Headaches. *Natural Medicine Journal* Vol.1: 2, March 1998.

Reader's Digest (ed.). *Magic and Medicine of Plants,* Fourth Edition. Pleasantville, NY: Reader's Digest Association, 1990.

Schultz, Stacey. The Dangers of Self-Dosing. *U.S. News & World Report,* July 13, 1998.

Werbach, Melvin R. *Nutritional Influences on Illness,* Second Edition. Tarzana, CA: Third Line Press, 1993.

Zubay, Geoffrey. *Biochemistry,* Second Edition. New York: Macmillan Publishing Co., 1988.

INDEX

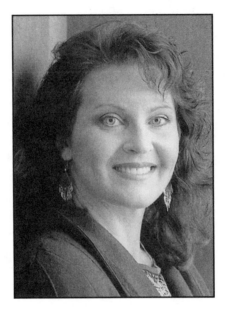

ABOUT THE AUTHOR

Dr. Eva Urbaniak is director of Alternative Medical Arts Associates, a center for natural healing located in Seattle, Washington. She received a Doctorate of Naturopathic Medicine from Bastyr University, and also holds degrees in human health sciences, psychology, and counseling. Dr. Urbaniak is a regular contributor to the *Well Being Journal*, and she is the author of *Healing Your Prostate: Natural Cures That Work* (Harbor Press, 1999). She speaks and writes extensively on the use of natural treatments to achieve optimal health and well being.

Photograph by Guy Kramer, Mukilteo, Washington